How Many CALORIES?
How Much FAT?

How Many CALORIES? How Much ∿∿∿∿∿ FAT?

*Guide to Calculating
the Nutritional Content
of the Foods You Eat*

*Rosemary Baskin
and the Editors of
Consumer Reports Books*

*Consumer Reports Books
A Division of Consumers Union
Yonkers, New York*

Published by Consumers Union of United States, Inc., Yonkers, New York 10703.

Library of Congress Cataloging-in-Publication Data
Baskin, Rosemary M.
    How many calories? how much fat? : guide to calculating the
nutritional content of the foods you eat / Rosemary Baskin and the
editors of Consumer Reports Books.
        p.   cm.
    Includes bibliographical references (p.   ).
    ISBN 0–89043–421–2
    1. Food—Fat content—Tables.   2. Food—Caloric content—Tables.
I. Consumer Reports Books.
TX551.B27   1991
641.1′4—dc20   91-34719
                                                                        CIP

Design by Tammy O'Bradovich

First printing, December 1991

Manufactured in the United States of America

How Many Calories? How Much Fat? is a Consumer Reports Book published by Consumers Union, the nonprofit organization that publishes *Consumer Reports,* the monthly magazine of test reports, product Ratings, and buying guidance. Established in 1936, Consumers Union is chartered under the Not-For-Profit Corporation Law of the State of New York.

The purposes of Consumers Union, as stated in its charter, are to provide consumers with information and counsel on consumer goods and services, to give information on all matters relating to the expenditure of the family income, and to initiate and to cooperate with individual and group efforts seeking to create and maintain decent living standards.

Consumers Union derives its income solely from the sale of *Consumer Reports* and other publications. In addition, expenses of occasional public service efforts may be met, in part, by nonrestrictive, noncommercial contributions, grants, and fees. Consumers Union accepts no advertising or product samples and is not beholden in any way to any commercial interest. Its Ratings and reports are solely for the use of the readers of its publications. Neither the Ratings nor the reports nor any Consumers Union publications, including this book, may be used in advertising or for any commercial purpose. Consumers Union will take all steps open to it to prevent such uses of its materials, its name, or the name of *Consumer Reports.*

～ CONTENTS

How Many CALORIES?
How Much FAT?

~ INTRODUCTION

~ Healthy eating has become a major topic of conversation for the 1990s; discussions everywhere include diet and cholesterol levels. Whether you are on a special diet or are just interested in good nutrition, this guide is intended as an aid in comparing foods and choosing those best for your needs. It lists available nutritional information about hundreds of food items and will enable you to analyze your own recipes with an eye to making them more healthful.

RDAS AND U.S. RDAS

Recommended Dietary Allowances (RDAs) were introduced in 1943 and have been revised about every five years and published by the National Academy of Sciences. They are recommendations—not requirements—developed by an appointed committee of nutrition scientists, and they are based on food surveys of people consuming a typical American diet. RDAs are designed to meet the nutritional needs of large groups of healthy people (not individuals) over a period of time (not necessarily daily). A large extra amount is added as a margin of safety, meaning that most individuals will not require even the RDA.

Since the typical American diet on which RDAs are based already contains excessive protein, fat, and refined foods—even before the "margin of safety" is added—it is questionable whether using the RDAs encourages a healthful way of eating. RDAs based on the typical American diet are inappropriate for anyone on a vegetarian diet (especially one that uses no animal protein, including dairy or egg products); the requirements for many vitamins and minerals would be different. The set of recommendations used by the World Health Organization would be more useful; they are based more on the eating patterns of populations using less animal protein and more complex carbohydrates.

The U.S. RDA was established by the U.S. Food and Drug Administration (FDA) specifically for use on food labels. Although RDAs are broken down into recommendations for different age and gender categories, there is no room on a food label to list recommendations for each one. To ensure that the product is evaluated according to the perceived needs of anyone consuming it, the U.S. RDAs on labels were created for each nutrient by taking the highest RDA of all categories (except pregnant or lactating women). They are therefore even more inflated than the RDAs.

The FDA is proposing the creation of new reference values called RDIs (Reference Daily Intake), which would replace the current U.S. RDAs and would represent the needs of a target group rather than those of the group with the highest needs. This would reflect a shift from a focus on nutritional inadequacies to a concern with excesses that have been linked to health problems.

FOOD COUNT GUIDE LISTINGS

The listings include calories, total fat and the portions that are saturated and polyunsaturated, calories from fat, cholesterol, sodium, potassium, protein, total carbohydrate, dietary fiber and sugars where available, calcium, iron, vitamin A, and vitamin C. The information has been gathered primarily from United States Department of Agriculture (USDA) reference books, and also from manufacturers and food labels. Information from a source other than the food label has been adjusted according to USDA regulations for food labeling so that all the information is presented consistently. These regulations prescribe a rounding off process in listing amounts in order to enable the consumer to calculate more easily. The following list explains how this is done:

Calories: up to and including 20 calories—rounded to the nearest 2 calories; from 20 up to and including 50 calories—rounded to the nearest 5 calories; above 50 calories—rounded to the nearest 10 calories.

Fat, Cholesterol, Protein, and Carbohydrate: rounded to the nearest gram or mg, unless less than 1.

Sodium, Potassium: less than 5 mg—rounded to 0; from 5 up to and including 140 mg—rounded to the nearest 5 mg; above 140 mg—rounded to the nearest 10 mg.

Percentage of U.S. RDA: from 0 up to and including 10 percent—rounded to the nearest 2 percent; from 10 percent up to and including 50 percent—rounded to the nearest 5 percent; above 50 percent—rounded to the nearest 10 percent.

Regulations are not stipulated for fiber or for sugars; listings are scarce for both. Where available, sugars are rounded to the nearest gram, unless less than 1. Fiber has been rounded to the nearest tenth of a gram, since the total you may be monitoring is a relatively small number.

"N.A." indicates that information for that listing was not available. When the listing includes more than one variety of the item, the value listed is an average of the varieties available.

Because amounts have been rounded off and adjusted, it should be clear that monitoring your nutritional intake can only be approximated and should not be approached as a precise laboratory exercise. Even the precise values given for foods in reference books may be based on the laboratory analysis of relatively few samples of the food. They could be different if the food were grown in another area or harvested at a different time. Thus assigning too precise a value is not justified, and rounding gives a useful estimate.

2 ∿

LABELING

Labeling of most foods is overseen by two government agencies. The USDA inspects and has labeling policies for most meat and poultry products and most eggs. It also grades many products (rates them for appearance, taste, texture, but not nutritional value). The FDA has regulations for labels on most other food products; it does no grading. There is overlap between the two agencies and sorting out what each does is very complicated. Moreover, there are many changes proposed for the new food labeling due to take effect in 1993. Regardless of where the policy originates, it is important to understand the meaning of the information on the label as it now appears.

TYPES OF INFORMATION ON A LABEL

There are two types of information on a food label—a list of ingredients and nutritional information per serving. Currently only the list of ingredients is required, except for some foods with standardized ingredients, such as ice cream. These foods have a "standard of identity" fixed by law and cannot use the product name unless they contain the ingredients specified in the description. The standardized food may just be listed by name on the label without specifying its ingredients. Some items, such as flavorings, may have their ingredients protected from competitors, and would thus appear on the label only as "flavoring." If you have allergies or special dietary needs and require more information than appears on the label, call or write the manufacturer. Many have toll-free numbers listed on the label.

The second type of information, nutritional information per serving, has generally been voluntary. It is required only if a nutrient is added to the food (e.g., fortification) or if a nutritional claim appears on the label or in advertising. Currently about half of packaged and processed foods carry voluntary nutrition information. A standard format includes serving size, servings per container, calories, protein, total carbohydrate, total fat, sodium, and percentage of U.S. RDA for protein and several vitamins and minerals. While some of this information was appropriate when concern focused on adequate amounts of nutrients, consumers now want to use label information to avoid excesses rather than to prevent deficiencies.

NEW FOOD LABELING LEGISLATION

A new food labeling bill was enacted in November 1990. If the legislative process proceeds on schedule, final regulations on how the new labeling will be implemented should be decided by November 1992 and new labeling will be in place by May 1993. The law will make nutritional information labeling mandatory for most foods under FDA jurisdiction and will focus on making it consistent with current knowledge of diet and health. Labels will still include serving size, servings per container, calories, protein, total fat, total carbohydrate, and sodium. The percentage of U.S. RDA for protein and the various vitamins and minerals will be dropped, since these are no longer of public health concern. Saturated fat, cholesterol, complex carbohydrate, sugar, and dietary fiber will be added. Various health groups have recommended that more information—such as calories from fat, unsaturated fat, calcium, and iron—be included. Whether these or others are added will depend on the outcome of hearings conducted during the period before final regulations are implemented.

WHAT TO LOOK FOR IN AN INGREDIENT LISTING

Ingredients are listed in descending order (the component that weighs most is listed first, etc.). Ingredients making up 2 percent or less of the food are listed at the end in random order. If you are concerned about the total amount of fats, sugars, or sodium, you must look at everything in the list to see where sources of these things may be hiding.

SOURCES OF FAT

Unsaturated fats are usually liquid at room temperature. They include:

- monounsaturated fats—olive, peanut, canola oils
- polyunsaturated fats—corn, cottonseed, safflower, soybean, sunflower, sesame oils.

Saturated fats are solid at room temperature, with the exception of the tropical oils (coconut, palm, palm kernel). Ingredients high in saturated fat include animal fat (lard), butter, cocoa butter, tropical oils, cream, egg yolk solids, hydrogenated vegetable oil, and vegetable shortening.

Hydrogenation converts unsaturated fats into saturated ones; it is done to make the fat more solid and to increase shelf life.

On food labels, "and/or" is often used in a list of fats. This doesn't tell you what was actually used; it merely lists the possible fats the manufacturer may have used.

SOURCES OF CARBOHYDRATE

Total carbohydrates include:

- simple carbohydrates (sugars)
- complex carbohydrates (whole grain products, beans, potatoes, cereals, other starches)
- dietary fiber (soluble and insoluble)—fiber is considered a complex carbohydrate, but furnishes no calories.

Dietary Fiber: Look for whole grains, legumes, bran, nuts, fruits, and vegetables. Breads with ingredients such as "whole wheat" or "100% whole wheat" are higher in fiber than those whose first ingredient is "wheat flour."

Sugars: These include sucrose (table sugar), beet or cane sugar, invert sugar, lactose, maltose, fructose, dextrose, high-fructose corn syrup, corn syrup, honey, molasses, and concentrated fruit juices.

Sorbitol, mannitol, and xylitol are sugar alcohols—sugars with the same number of calories but with slower absorption by the body; products containing these may be labeled "sugarless" or "no sugar." Saccharin, aspartame, and acesulfame-K are artificial sweeteners.

SOURCES OF SODIUM

In addition to salt (sodium chloride), look for anything with "sodium" as part of the name. Items like broths, soy sauce, Worcestershire sauce, MSG (monosodium glutamate), and baking soda are hidden sources of sodium.

FOOD ADDITIVES

Anything added in processing is by definition an intentional additive. Additives may also be indirectly added—for example, the residues from drugs fed to animals, which would not, of course, show up on an ingredients list. Most intentional additives are present in small enough amounts that they are included only at the end of the list. About three thousand additives have been approved for use in the United States. Here are some of the more common ones you will encounter, and the reasons they are used:

- Sodium or calcium propionate, sodium benzoate, potassium sorbate, nitrites, nitrates, sugar, salt—prevent bacterial growth, protect color or flavor.
- Sodium sulfite, sulfur dioxide, sodium and potassium bisulfite, sodium and potassium metabisulfite—prevent spoilage and browning of foods. Because of problems with allergic reactions, restrictions have been placed on the use of sulfites in supervised products; however, sulfites may be present even though not listed if they are part of a product with a standard of identity.
- BHA (butylated hydroxyanisole), BHT (butylated hydroxytoluene), EDTA (ethylene diamine tetraacetic acid), vitamin E—prevent spoilage.
- Ascorbic acid (vitamin C), citric acid—prevent browning of fruits and vegetables.
- Other vitamins and minerals (calcium, iron)—fortification or enrichment.
- Gums, pectin, carrageenan, starch, gelatin—thickeners.
- Calcium silicate, silicon dioxide—keep salts and powders from caking.
- Lactic acid, sodium citrate, calcium lactate, acetic acid (vinegar)—control acidity.
- Color additives—certified colors have initials and a number (FD&C Red No. 2); uncertified colors include things like beet juice or paprika.

There are additives which we don't usually think of as additives, such as sweeteners (sugars, honey, molasses) or extenders (vegetable or plant proteins). If they are present in large enough amounts, they are considered ingredients.

SOME TERMS USED ON LABELS

Serving Size: A reasonable quantity used by an adult. Check this when comparing products to make sure you are using similar amounts. One brand may give information for a teaspoon, while another does so for a tablespoon. Information for canned soups is often given for an 8-oz serving (1 cup), yet the can contains 1½ to 1¾ servings.

Serving size is now determined by the manufacturer, and there is no consistency. The FDA has proposed standard serving sizes in 159 food categories.

Dietetic: At least one ingredient has been changed or restricted.

Reduced Calorie: At least one third fewer calories than the original.

Low Calorie: No more than 40 calories per serving. If the food is naturally low in calories, it cannot have this designation immediately before the name, because this would imply the food had been changed to lower calories.

Lowfat/Low Fat/Lean/Extra Lean: "Lowfat" applies only to milk products with fat content 0.5 to 2 percent by weight. "Low fat" and "lean" can be used only on meat with no more than 10 percent fat by weight. "Extra lean" means the meat has no more than 5 percent by weight. However, ground beef and hamburger have a different designation: "lean" or "extra lean" can be used if the fat content is no more than 22.5 percent by weight (the standard for regular hamburger is 30 percent).

Percent Fat Free: This does not mean that the stated percentage of fat has been removed, but rather that this percentage is not fat. To avoid confusion the percentage of fat by weight is also listed. It also does not mean that this is the percentage of calories from fat. Four ounces of a meat that is 80 percent fat free (20 percent fat by weight) and that contains 300 calories would have 200 calories from fat (67 percent of calories).

Reduced Cholesterol: The proposed FDA regulation would allow the term "reduced cholesterol" for foods with at least 75 percent less cholesterol than the original product.

Low Cholesterol: The USDA considers "low cholesterol" a suitable label on food with 20 mg per 3.5-oz serving. The label must list nutritional information if a cholesterol claim appears on it. A proposed FDA regulation would allow a "low cholesterol" label for 20 mg or less per serving, provided the food also met the fat requirements for "cholesterol free."

Cholesterol Free/No Cholesterol: Some foods using these terms never had any cholesterol, because only foods of animal origin contain it. Currently foods do not have to meet any fat requirements to use this label. A proposed FDA regulation would allow the use of these terms for foods with fewer than 2 mg cholesterol per serving, but the food could not have more than 5 grams of total fat and 2 grams of saturated fat per serving.

Unsalted/No Salt Added: Foods processed without salt that are usually processed with salt.

Reduced Sodium: At least 75 percent less sodium than the original product.

Low Sodium: No more than 140 mg per serving. Some products with several food components (e.g., a frozen dinner) can have an average of 140 mg per component, so a product with five components could have up to 700 mg sodium and still be called "low sodium."

Very Low Sodium: No more than 35 mg per serving.

Sodium Free: Less than 5 mg per serving.

No Added Sugar: Usually a product sweetened with a naturally occurring sweetener such as fruit or fruit juice.

Sugar Free/No Sugar: Usually low calorie or reduced in calories. Otherwise the food must have another purpose, such as a food using sorbitol as a sweetener in a diabetic diet—the calories are the same, but the food is useful because it is absorbed more slowly.

Lite/Light: For meat or poultry products, this usually means that a product has 25 percent fewer calories than the original; however, it can also mean less fat, sodium, or breading. On other products it can also mean such things as lighter color or texture. The FDA is preparing a definition.

Natural: Usually means that a product has been produced with no intentional additives. However, the FDA has no regulation for "natural" and although the USDA has a general policy, each product is reviewed separately.

No Preservatives: Can be used only on USDA-regulated foods that would be expected to contain preservatives and do not. It does not mean "no additives." There is no FDA definition, so it has no meaning when used on FDA products.

FAT INTAKE

When monitoring fat intake, the two things to pay most attention to are total fat and the amount of fat that is saturated. This is not to say that watching your cholesterol intake is not important—excessive amounts should be avoided—but all indications are that total fat is at least as important and that the saturated component is the worst culprit in raising blood cholesterol.

Keeping the saturated component as low as possible will increase the polyunsaturated and monounsaturated fats in what you do eat, and keeping total fat as low as possible will in itself help to regulate cholesterol intake. Virtually all health care organizations agree that no more than 30 percent of the day's calories should come from fat; many advise less than that. No more than one-third of the total fat should come from saturated fats. Polyunsaturated fats should also contribute no more than one-third of the total fat. Monounsaturated sources make up the remainder. The recommendation is to stress the use of monounsaturated fats while keeping saturated fats to a minimum, meanwhile keeping an eye on the total.

Listings for monounsaturated fat, which are not plentiful, are not included here, but they can be estimated by subtracting the sum of the saturated and polyunsaturated fats from the total fat. All fats contain a mixture of saturated, monounsaturated, and polyunsaturated fatty acids. A look at the table listings for oils will show you which are the richest sources for each type of fat.

CALORIES FROM FAT

The percentage of calories from fat is currently listed on some food labels and has become popular in judging a food's fat content. Many people, however, mis-interpret the 30 percent goal to mean that every food item should meet it, rather than the total for the day. While percentages are helpful in comparing similar foods, they can be misleading unless you keep in mind the actual amount of fat and calories involved. One food containing 50 calories and 3 grams of fat and a second food containing 700 calories and 42 grams of fat both have 54 percent of their calories from fat; however, the first has 27 calories from fat, while the second has 378 calories from fat. Comparing the percentages is not as helpful as noting the actual contribution from fat.

Because of the misleading possibilities in using the percentage of calories from fat, the American Dietetic Association has recommended that the number of calories from fat be included when new labeling regulations take effect. Ac-cordingly, this guide lists the calories from fat, rounded in the same way as total calories.

MONITORING FAT INTAKE

An easy way to monitor fat intake is to determine the number of calories from fat that is your upper goal limit, and make choices that keep the total within that limit. For someone whose typical intake is about 2000 calories a day, 30 percent of the calories would be about 600 calories. These 600 calories from fat should be divided among saturated, polyunsaturated, and monounsaturated sources. You can determine your approximate calorie and fat intake by keeping a food diary for two or three typical days and using this book to add up your totals. You will be able to determine the total number of calories from fat directly from the listings. Since the saturated and polyunsaturated components are listed in grams, multiply the grams by 9 (fat contains 9 calories per gram) to determine the number of calories from that fat, and compare the totals with the recommended limit to see where you may need to make changes in your diet. Remember that the projected intake is an upper limit goal, and that it is an approximation.

If you prefer to count the number of grams of fat, the 600 calories from fat allowed in the example above would translate to about 67 grams of fat (600 ÷ 9 = 66.7). You could then compare how much of that was coming from each type of fat.

CHOLESTEROL

Controversy still exists regarding whether dietary cholesterol intake needs to be limited for everyone, but health organizations regard it as prudent to limit cholesterol to 300 mg a day or less. Remember that cholesterol is found only in foods from animal sources. Therefore, foods such as vegetable-oil margarines and peanut butter can have no cholesterol but still be high in fat.

SODIUM AND POTASSIUM

The recommendation for sodium intake is 3000 mg a day or less; people with health problems that respond to a lower intake should follow the recommendation appropriate for them. The estimated minimum sodium requirement for healthy persons is only 500 mg per day, according to the tenth edition of the RDAs released in 1989. This is a marked decrease from the estimated "safe and adequate daily intake" of 1100 to 3300 mg in 1980.

Potassium values are useful for those who need to monitor intake because of losses from diuretics or other health considerations. The estimated minimum requirement for healthy adults is 2000 mg per day, with the caution that the most desirable intake may be in the area of 3500 mg per day. As with sodium, the intake should be adjusted for those with special needs.

PROTEIN

The RDA recommendation for protein is 45 grams for women and 56 grams for men (this varies with age and size). Most Americans consume more protein than necessary (sometimes two to three times what is needed), and this has been linked to calcium depletion from bone, increased incidence of breast and colon cancer, and increased stress on the kidneys.

CARBOHYDRATE AND FIBER

There is no RDA recommendation for total carbohydrate intake but *Consumer Reports* recommends that about 55 percent of calories come from carbohydrates. In any case, decreased fat intake will result in increased consumption of carbohydrates. Total carbohydrate is a combination of simple carbohydrate (sugar), complex carbohydrate (starch), and dietary fiber (soluble and insoluble). Fiber and sugar content are listed here when they are available.

Although there is no consensus on the recommended amount of fiber, it is agreed that most Americans do not consume enough. One suggested goal is 20 to 35 grams a day. Data on soluble and insoluble fiber has not been agreed on by fiber researchers; indeed, the methods for determining amounts of dietary fiber have not been standardized.

The values available here are for total dietary fiber (including both soluble and insoluble). Fiber listings on food labels should become more available as the new label regulations requiring them take effect. In general, whole grains are good sources of insoluble fiber, while legumes and oat bran are good sources of soluble fiber; fruits (with edible seeds and/or peel) provide both.

CALCIUM, IRON, VITAMIN A, AND VITAMIN C

Calcium, iron, vitamin A, and vitamin C are listed as a percentage of the U.S. RDA, as they are currently on food labels. Because the RDAs (and therefore the U.S.

RDAs) are not meant to be applied to individuals, the percentages listed should be used to evaluate a food as a good or poor source of the nutrient, but not as a measurement for meeting an individual's specific requirements.

CALCULATING RECIPES

Calculating nutritional values for your own recipes is quite easy to do. Look up the recipe ingredients in the tables and list them, multiplying or dividing to fit your recipe. For example, if your recipe calls for 2½ cups of flour, and the table gives values for 1 cup, multiply the table values by 2.5. Add up the totals for the values you are interested in, and divide by the number of portions you will use. This gives you the nutritional information per serving. To calculate the calories from fat, multiply the grams of fat by 9 (fat supplies 9 calories per gram). For values listed as less than 1 ("<1"), use 0.5 for your estimate; for percentages of U.S. RDAs listed as less than 2 percent ("*"), use 1 percent for your estimate. Remember that the values are rounded; all you need is a ballpark figure.

Knowledge about your food choices is essential to making good ones; it is hoped this guide will help.

~ FOOD COUNT
GUIDE CHECKLIST

RECOMMENDED DAILY GOALS

☐ **TOTAL FAT:**   No more than 30 percent of day's total calories. (Many health professionals recommend less than this.)

☐ **SATURATED FAT:**   Up to ⅓ of total fat.

☐ **POLYUNSATURATED FAT:**   Up to ⅓ of total fat.

☐ **MONOUNSATURATED FAT:**   At least ⅓ of total fat.

☐ **CHOLESTEROL:**   300 mg per day or less.

☐ **SODIUM:**   Estimated minimum requirement for healthy individuals is 500 mg per day. Recommended intake is no more than 3000 mg per day for healthy individuals; appropriate levels for health problems should be followed.

☐ **POTASSIUM:**   Estimated minimum requirement for healthy individuals is 2000 mg per day; desirable intake may be more in area of 3500 mg per day. As with sodium, intake should be adjusted for those with special needs.

☐ **PROTEIN:**   Recommended intake varies with sex, age, and weight. Most Americans consume more than needed.

☐ **FIBER:**   No consensus on recommended amount; one suggested amount is 20 to 35 grams per day.

☐ **CALCIUM, IRON, VITAMIN A, AND VITAMIN C:**   Currently listed on food labels as percentages of U.S. RDA. May be replaced by new value (RDI) or may not be included on labels at all, depending on results of hearings on new label regulations due to take effect in May 1993. Use to evaluate a food as a good or poor source of the nutrient.

∿BEVERAGES

∿ This section is divided into nonalcoholic and alcoholic beverages. Fiber content of beverages is negligible; values for sugar content are given where available.

~ BEVERAGES, NONALCOHOLIC	Calories	Saturated fat (g)	Polyunsaturated fat (g)	Total fat (g)	Calories from fat	Cholesterol (mg)
Clam and tomato juice, canned, 5.5-oz can	80	0	0	<1	N.A.	N.A.
Club soda, carbonated, 12 oz	0	0	0	0	0	0
Coffee, brewed, 6 oz	4	0	0	0	0	0
instant, 1 tsp powder	4	0	0	0	0	0
instant flavored powder, 2 tsp	60	3	0	3	25	N.A.
sugar-free varieties	35	N.A.	N.A.	2	20	0
Coffee substitute Postum, 6 oz, all varieties	12	N.A.	N.A.	0	0	0
Eggnog and eggnog-flavored mix (see Dairy Products & Eggs)						
Frostee flavored drink, 1 cup, all varieties	190	N.A.	N.A.	8	70	N.A.
Fruit-flavored drink powder, 1 cup prepared	100	0	0	0	0	0
sugar-free, 8 oz, all varieties	4	N.A.	N.A.	0	0	0
canned, 1 cup	110	0	0	0	0	0
frozen, 1 cup prepared	110	0	0	0	0	0
Fruit juices (see Fruits & Fruit Juices)						
Fruit-juice drink, frozen, 1 cup prepared	120	<1	<1	<1	N.A.	0
Lemonade, frozen concentrate, 1 cup prepared	100	0	0	<1	N.A.	0
Milk and milk drinks (see Dairy Products & Eggs)						
Orange drink, canned, 6 oz	90	0	0	0	0	0
Orange-flavored drink, breakfast type, frozen concentrate with pulp, 6 oz prepared	90	0	<1	<1	N.A.	0
with orange juice and pulp	80	0	0	0	0	0
powder, 3 tsp	90	<1	0	0	0	0

*Less than 2% U.S. RDA

Sodium (mg)	Potassium (mg)	Protein (g)	Carbohy-drate (g)	Sugars (g)	Calcium (% U.S. RDA)	Iron (% U.S. RDA)	Vitamin A (% U.S. RDA)	Vitamin C (% U.S. RDA)
660	150	1	18	N.A.	2	6	8	10
75	5	0	0	N.A.	*	N.A.	*	*
0	95	<1	<1	N.A.	*	4	N.A.	*
0	65	<1	<1	N.A.	*	*	*	*
65	130	<1	9	7	*	*	*	*
50	190	0	3	<1	*	*	*	*
0	95	0	3	<1	*	*	*	*
160	240	2	29	N.A.	2	6	*	*
40	0	0	25	28	4	*	*	50
15	20	0	0	N.A.	*	*	*	10
55	60	<1	29	27	*	4	*	120
10	30	<1	29	25	*	*	*	180
10	190	<1	30	18	*	4	*	25
10	40	<1	26	22	*	2	*	15
30	35	0	24	17	*	4	*	110
15	230	0	23	24	6	*	*	210
20	250	<1	21	N.A.	20	*	*	170
0	40	0	24	26	4	*	30	160

~ BEVERAGES, NONALCOHOLIC/ ALCOHOLIC	Calories	Saturated fat (g)	Polyunsat-urated fat (g)	Total fat (g)	Calories from fat	Choles-terol (mg)
Soda, carbonated, 12 oz, all flavors	160	N.A.	N.A.	0	0	0
low-calorie, with saccharin, 12 oz, all flavors	2	0	0	0	0	0
Tea, brewed, 6 oz	2	0	0	0	0	0
instant lemon-flavored, with saccharin, 2 tsp	6	0	0	0	0	0
instant lemon-flavored, with sugar, 3 tsp	90	0	0	<1	N.A.	0
instant powder, 1 tsp	2	0	0	0	0	0
Thirst-quencher drink, bottled, 1 cup	60	0	0	<1	N.A.	0
Tonic water, carbonated, 12 oz	130	0	0	0	0	0
Water, bottled, Perrier, 1 cup	0	0	0	0	0	0
Beer, regular, 12-oz can	150	0	0	0	0	0
light, 12-oz can	100	0	0	0	0	0
Bloody Mary, 5 oz	120	0	0	<1	N.A.	0
Bourbon and soda, 4 oz	110	0	0	0	0	0
Coffee liqueur, 1.5 oz	170	0	0	<1	N.A.	0
Crème de menthe, 1.5 oz	190	0	0	<1	N.A.	0
Daiquiri, 2 oz	110	0	0	0	0	0
Gin and tonic, 7.5 oz	170	0	0	0	0	0
Manhattan, 2 oz	130	0	0	0	0	0
Martini, 2.5 oz	160	0	0	0	0	0
Piña colada, 4.5 oz	260	1	<1	3	25	0
Screwdriver, 7 oz	170	0	0	<1	N.A.	0
Spirits, distilled (gin, rum, vodka, whiskey) 1.5 oz jigger	100	0	0	0	0	0
Tequila sunrise, 5.5 oz	190	0	0	<1	N.A.	0

*Less than 2% U.S. RDA

Sodium (mg)	Potassium (mg)	Protein (g)	Carbohydrate (g)	Sugars (g)	Calcium (% U.S. RDA)	Iron (% U.S. RDA)	Vitamin A (% U.S. RDA)	Vitamin C (% U.S. RDA)
40	0	0	40	N.A.	*	*	*	*
55	5	<1	<1	N.A.	*	*	*	*
5	65	0	<1	0	*	*	*	*
15	40	<1	1	N.A.	*	*	*	*
N.A.	50	<1	22	N.A.	*	*	*	*
0	45	<1	<1	N.A.	*	*	*	*
95	25	0	15	14	*	*	*	*
15	0	0	32	N.A.	*	N.A.	*	*
0	0	0	0	N.A.	4	*	*	*
20	90	<1	13	4	*	*	*	*
10	65	<1	5	1	*	*	*	*
330	220	<1	5	N.A.	*	4	10	35
15	0	0	0	N.A.	*	N.A.	*	*
0	15	0	24	N.A.	*	*	*	*
0	0	0	21	N.A.	*	*	*	N.A.
0	15	0	4	N.A.	*	*	*	*
10	10	0	16	N.A.	*	N.A.	*	*
0	15	0	2	N.A.	*	*	N.A.	*
0	15	0	<1	N.A.	*	*	N.A.	*
10	100	<1	40	N.A.	*	2	*	10
0	330	1	18	N.A.	*	*	2	110
0	0	0	0	0	*	*	*	*
5	180	<1	15	N.A.	*	4	4	60

～ BEVERAGES, ALCOHOLIC

	Calories	Saturated fat (g)	Polyunsat- urated fat (g)	Total fat (g)	Calories from fat	Choles- terol (mg)
Tom Collins, 7.5 oz	120	0	0	0	0	0
Whiskey sour, 3 oz	120	0	0	<1	N.A.	0
Wine, sweet dessert, 2 oz	90	0	0	0	0	0
Wine, table, 3.5 oz, red, rosé, white	70	0	0	0	0	0

Sodium (mg)	Potassium (mg)	Protein (g)	Carbohy-drate (g)	Sugars (g)	Calcium (% U.S. RDA)	Iron (% U.S. RDA)	Vitamin A (% U.S. RDA)	Vitamin C (% U.S. RDA)
40	20	<1	3	N.A.	*	N.A.	*	6
10	50	<1	5	N.A.	*	*	*	20
5	55	<1	7	10	*	*	N.A.	*
10	90	<1	1	2	*	2	*	*

∿ BREADS

∿ BISCUITS

∿ PANCAKES

∿ & ROLLS

∿ *Values for sugar content are not widely available and so are not included here. Frozen pancakes, waffles, etc. that are part of a packaged meal are listed in the Frozen Breakfast Entree section of "Entrees and Side Dishes."*

~ BREADS, BISCUITS, PANCAKES & ROLLS	Calories	Saturated fat (g)	Polyunsat- urated fat (g)	Total fat (g)	Calories from fat	Choles- terol (mg)
Bagels						
Lender's, frozen, 2 oz (plain, egg [contains 5 mg choles- terol], garlic, onion)	160	N.A.	N.A.	1	10	0
2½ oz, blueberry, cinnamon raisin	200	N.A.	N.A.	1	10	0
soft original	210	N.A.	N.A.	3	25	10
3⅛ oz Big and Crusty (egg contains 20 mg cholesterol)	240	N.A.	N.A.	2	18	0
Sara Lee, frozen, 3 oz, all kinds (egg contains 20 mg cholesterol)	230	N.A.	N.A.	1	10	0
Baking powder and soda (see Grains, Pasta & Flour						
Biscuits						
Pillsbury, 1 biscuit, regular and Ballard Ovenready	50	0	0	1	10	0
1869 Brand, Big Country, Heat 'n Eat, Hungry Jack, 1 biscuit, all varieties	90	1	<1	4	35	<1
Bisquick (General Mills), ½ cup mix	240	2	1	8	70	0
Bread						
cinnamon raisin, Continen- tal, 1 slice	80	N.A.	N.A.	1	10	3
cracked wheat, Pepperidge Farm, 1 slice	70	N.A.	N.A.	1	10	N.A.
French, Pillsbury, 1″ slice, crusty	60	0	0	<1	N.A.	0
Italian, Wonder, 1 slice, family loaf	70	N.A.	N.A.	1	10	3
multigrain, Beefsteak, 1 slice	70	N.A.	N.A.	1	10	0
oatmeal goodness, Conti- nental, 1 slice	90	N.A.	N.A.	2	18	0

*Less than 2% U.S. RDA

Sodium (mg)	Potassium (mg)	Protein (g)	Carbohy-drate (g)	Sugars (g)	Calcium (% U.S. RDA)	Iron (% U.S. RDA)	Vitamin A (% U.S. RDA)	Vitamin C (% U.S. RDA)
330	N.A.	7	31	1.2	2	8	*	*
280	N.A.	8	39	1.4	*	10	2	*
350	N.A.	7	36	N.A.	*	10	*	*
430	N.A.	9	47	N.A.	2	15	*	*
490	N.A.	9	47	N.A.	*	15	*	*
180	105	1	10	N.A.	*	2	*	*
300	40	2	13	N.A.	*	4	*	*
700	80	4	37	N.A.	8	8	*	*
140	N.A.	2	15	0.6	2	4	*	*
140	N.A.	2	13	N.A.	*	4	*	*
120	15	2	11	N.A.	*	4	*	*
160	N.A.	2	13	0.7	4	6	*	*
130	N.A.	3	11	1.6	4	6	*	*
140	N.A.	4	15	1	4	6	*	*

～ BREADS, BISCUITS, PANCAKES & ROLLS	Calories	Saturated fat (g)	Polyunsaturated fat (g)	Total fat (g)	Calories from fat	Cholesterol (mg)
pita pocket, 1⅓ oz (1 whole pocket)	110	N.A.	N.A.	<1	N.A.	N.A.
pumpernickel, 1 slice	80	N.A.	N.A.	<1	N.A.	N.A.
rye, Beefsteak, 1 slice, all varieties	70	N.A.	N.A.	1	10	3
wheat or white, Wonder, 1 slice	70	N.A.	N.A.	1	10	3
light, 1 slice	40	0	0	0	0	0
whole wheat, Wonder, 100% whole wheat, 1 slice	70	N.A.	N.A.	1	10	3
Bread crumbs, Progresso, 2 tbsp plain (flavored varieties contain 280 mg sodium)	60	N.A.	N.A.	<1	N.A.	0
Bread sticks						
Pillsbury, Soft, 1 stick	100	<1	0	2	18	0
Stella D'Oro, 1 piece, plain, flavored (dietetic has <10 mg sodium)	45	N.A.	N.A.	1	10	0
Brown bread, B & M, ⅒ of 10-oz can, plain, raisin	90	0	0	0	0	0
Buns, hamburger (see Rolls, below)						
Coating mix						
French's chicken coating mix, ¼ pkg, BBQ, garlic butter, Italian parmesan	50	N.A.	N.A.	1	10	N.A.
fish coating mix, ¼ pkg, lemon dill	45	N.A.	N.A.	1	10	N.A.
Shake 'n Bake (General Foods), ¼ pouch, all varieties (does 2 pieces)	80	N.A.	N.A.	2	18	0
oven fry coating, ¼ pouch, all varieties	100	N.A.	N.A.	2	18	0
Corn Muffin mix, Robin Hood, pouch, ⅙ mix	130	N.A.	N.A.	2	18	N.A.
Cornbread mix, Ballard, ⅛ loaf	140	N.A.	N.A.	3	25	N.A.

*Less than 2% U.S. RDA

Sodium (mg)	Potassium (mg)	Protein (g)	Carbohy-drate (g)	Sugars (g)	Calcium (% U.S. RDA)	Iron (% U.S. RDA)	Vitamin A (% U.S. RDA)	Vitamin C (% U.S. RDA)
220	45	4	21	1	4	6	*	*
170	140	3	15	2.7	2	6	*	*
170	N.A.	3	13	0.8	4	6	*	*
140	N.A.	3	13	0.8	4	6	*	*
120	N.A.	3	7	2	4	4	*	*
160	N.A.	3	12	1.8	2	6	*	*
110	20	2	11	N.A.	2	2	*	*
230	20	3	17	N.A.	*	6	*	*
N.A.	N.A.	1	6	N.A.	N.A.	N.A.	N.A.	N.A.
340	160	2	22	2	4	4	*	*
380	N.A.	1	8	N.A.	2	2	*	4
270	N.A.	<1	7	N.A.	*	2	*	4
590	45	1	14	N.A.	*	*	4	*
820	40	2	19	N.A.	*	4	6	*
250	60	3	24	N.A.	*	6	2	*
570	75	3	25	N.A.	2	2	*	*

BREADS, BISCUITS, PANCAKES & ROLLS	Calories	Saturated fat (g)	Polyunsaturated fat (g)	Total fat (g)	Calories from fat	Cholesterol (mg)
Cornbread Twists, Pillsbury, 1 twist	70	1	0	4	35	5
Cream of tartar (*see* Grains, Pasta & Flour)						
Crispbread, Weight Watchers, 2 wafers, all kinds	30	0	0	0	0	N.A.
Croissant						
Dunkin' Donuts, 1 plain	310	N.A.	N.A.	19	170	0
almond, chocolate, 1 pastry	430	N.A.	N.A.	28	250	0
Pepperidge Farm all butter petite, 1 pastry	120	N.A.	N.A.	7	60	N.A.
Sandwich Quarters, 1 roll	180	N.A.	N.A.	9	80	N.A.
Sara Lee all butter, 1 pastry	170	N.A.	N.A.	9	80	N.A.
petite, 1 pastry	120	N.A.	N.A.	6	50	N.A.
Croutons, Pepperidge Farm, ½ oz, all varieties	70	N.A.	N.A.	3	25	N.A.
English muffin, Thomas', all varieties	130	N.A.	N.A.	1	10	0
Fillo dough, Apollo, 1 oz (number of sheets in 1 oz depends on size of sheets in pkg)	80	0	0	0	0	0
Flours (*see* Grains, Pasta & Flour)						
French toast, frozen (*see* Entrees & Side Dishes)						
Fruit bread, Pillsbury Quick Mix, ¹⁄₁₂ loaf, all varieties	170	N.A.	N.A.	5	45	N.A.
Matzo crackers, Manischewitz, 1 oz, all varieties (whole wheat with bran contains 6 gm dietary fiber; egg 'n onion contains 15 mg cholesterol)	110	0	<1	<1	N.A.	0
Melba toast, Devonsheer, ½ oz (3 slices)	50	N.A.	N.A.	<1	N.A.	0

*Less than 2% U.S. RDA

Sodium (mg)	Potassium (mg)	Protein (g)	Carbohy-drate (g)	Sugars (g)	Calcium (% U.S. RDA)	Iron (% U.S. RDA)	Vitamin A (% U.S. RDA)	Vitamin C (% U.S. RDA)
140	15	2	8	N.A.	*	2	*	*
55	N.A.	<1	7	N.A.	*	*	*	*
240	N.A.	7	27	2	N.A.	N.A.	N.A.	N.A.
250	N.A.	8	38	3	N.A.	N.A.	N.A.	N.A.
160	N.A.	3	13	N.A.	4	6	*	*
240	N.A.	4	20	N.A.	2	6	6	*
240	N.A.	4	19	N.A.	2	8	6	*
160	N.A.	3	13	N.A.	*	4	4	*
190	N.A.	2	9	N.A.	*	2	*	*
210	N.A.	4	26	2.5	6	6	*	*
100	25	3	18	N.A.	N.A.	N.A.	N.A.	N.A.
170	55	3	29	N.A.	2	4	*	*
0	40	4	23	6	N.A.	8	*	*
90	N.A.	2	12	N.A.	*	4	*	*

~ BREADS, BISCUITS, PANCAKES & ROLLS	Calories	Saturated fat (g)	Polyunsaturated fat (g)	Total fat (g)	Calories from fat	Cholesterol (mg)
Muffins (*see* Desserts)						
Pancakes						
batter, frozen, Aunt Jemima, 3.6 oz, all varieties	190	<1	<1	3	25	25
frozen entrees (*see* Entrees & Side Dishes)						
Microwave						
Aunt Jemima, original, blueberry, buttermilk, 3 pancakes (3.48 oz)	210	<1	<1	3	25	20
lite buttermilk	140	N.A.	N.A.	3	25	N.A.
mixes						
Aunt Jemima, three 4″ pancakes, original flavor	200	N.A.	N.A.	7	60	65
complete	250	<1	<1	4	35	15
Aunt Jemima, three 4″ pancakes, buttermilk	190	N.A.	N.A.	3	25	N.A.
complete	230	<1	<1	3	25	15
Bisquick Shake 'n Pour, three 4″ pancakes, original, apple cinnamon, blueberry, buttermilk	270	N.A.	N.A.	5	45	0
oat bran	240	N.A.	N.A.	4	35	0
Pizza crust, Pillsbury All Ready, ⅛ of crust	90	<1	<1	1	10	0
Rolls						
brown 'n serve, Wonder, 1 oz, gem style, buttermilk	80	N.A.	N.A.	2	18	3
French rolls du jour, 3½ oz	230	N.A.	N.A.	2	18	0
Italian crusty rolls, 1¼ oz	80	N.A.	N.A.	1	10	0
crescent, Pillsbury, 1 roll	100	2	0	6	50	5
dinner						
Pepperidge Farm, finger or old-fashioned, 1 roll	60	N.A.	N.A.	2	18	N.A.

*Less than 2% U.S. RDA

Sodium (mg)	Potassium (mg)	Protein (g)	Carbohy-drate (g)	Sugars (g)	Calcium (% U.S. RDA)	Iron (% U.S. RDA)	Vitamin A (% U.S. RDA)	Vitamin C (% U.S. RDA)
740	110	5	37	1.8	6	10	*	*
830	125	6	41	1.8	15	15	*	*
660	50	7	28	N.A.	20	12	*	*
590	170	7	28	1.4	20	10	4	*
1020	190	7	50	2.1	10	15	N.A.	N.A.
810	90	5	37	1.3	15	6	*	*
950	220	7	46	2	30	15	*	*
860	110	6	49	N.A.	10	10	*	*
580	170	7	45	1	8	10	*	*
170	20	3	16	N.A.	*	6	*	*
140	N.A.	2	13	0.6	4	4	*	*
490	N.A.	9	45	1.8	15	30	*	*
200	N.A.	3	16	0.6	6	8	*	*
230	65	2	11	N.A.	*	2	*	*
90	N.A.	2	8	N.A.	2	2	*	*

~ BREADS, BISCUITS, PANCAKES & ROLLS	Calories	Saturated fat (g)	Polyunsat-urated fat (g)	Total fat (g)	Calories from fat	Choles-terol (mg)
Pillsbury, 1 roll, butterflake	140	2	<1	5	45	5
hot, Pillsbury mix, 1 roll	120	N.A.	N.A.	2	18	N.A.
frankfurter						
Pepperidge Farm, 1 roll	140	N.A.	N.A.	3	25	N.A.
Wonder, 1 oz	80	N.A.	N.A.	1	10	3
light, 1½ oz	80	N.A.	N.A.	1	10	3
hamburger, Wonder, 1.5 oz	120	N.A.	N.A.	2	18	3
sandwich, Pepperidge Farm, 1 roll	160	N.A.	N.A.	3	25	N.A.
Stuffing mix, ½ cup prepared, all varieties, regular or microwave	180	N.A.	N.A.	9	80	15
Toast-r cakes, Thomas', 1 cake, all varieties	110	N.A.	N.A.	3	25	N.A.
Tortilla						
corn, Old El Paso, 1 shell	60	N.A.	N.A.	1	10	N.A.
flour, 1 shell	150	N.A.	N.A.	3	25	N.A.
taco or tostada shell, Old El Paso, 1 shell	60	N.A.	N.A.	3	25	0
Waffles						
Aunt Jemima, frozen, 2 waffles, original, apple-cinnamon, blueberry, butter-milk	180	1	<1	6	50	6
wholegrain wheat, oat-bran, 2 waffles	150	N.A.	N.A.	3	25	0
Downyflake, frozen, 2 waf-fles, regular	120	N.A.	N.A.	3	25	0
blueberry, buttermilk, hot-n-buttery, jumbo regular, 2 waffles	180	N.A.	N.A.	5	45	0
rice bran, 2 waffles	210	N.A.	N.A.	11	100	0
multigrain, oat bran, Roman meal, 2 waffles	260	N.A.	N.A.	14	130	0

*Less than 2% U.S. RDA

Sodium (mg)	Potassium (mg)	Protein (g)	Carbohydrate (g)	Sugars (g)	Calcium (% U.S. RDA)	Iron (% U.S. RDA)	Vitamin A (% U.S. RDA)	Vitamin C (% U.S. RDA)
520	30	3	20	N.A.	*	6	*	*
220	45	4	21	N.A.	*	6	2	*
320	N.A.	5	23	N.A.	4	6	*	*
150	N.A.	2	14	0.6	4	4	*	*
210	N.A.	5	13	4	6	8	*	*
230	N.A.	4	21	0.9	6	8	*	*
240	N.A.	5	27	N.A.	6	10	*	*
620	75	4	21	N.A.	2	6	6	*
180	40	2	18	N.A.	*	*	*	*
170	35	1	10	0.5	2	*	*	*
360	N.A.	4	27	N.A.	2	10	*	*
60	20	<1	6	0.5	*	*	*	*
500	95	4	29	1.5	15	20	*	*
680	180	6	29	3	20	40	*	*
420	50	3	20	N.A.	*	10	*	*
600	75	4	30	N.A.	*	20	*	*
230	125	5	25	3.5	6	25	*	*
590	160	6	30	3.2	6	30	*	*

~ BREADS, BISCUITS, PANCAKES & ROLLS	Calories	Saturated fat (g)	Polyunsat-urated fat (g)	Total fat (g)	Calories from fat	Choles-terol (mg)
Eggo, frozen, 1 waffle, all varieties (nutrigrain and oat bran varieties contain 0 mg cholesterol)	130	1	1	5	45	10
Waffle, Belgian						
Belgian Chef, frozen, 1 waffle	90	N.A.	N.A.	3	25	0
Weight Watchers, frozen, 1 waffle	120	2	<1	4	35	5
Yeasts (see Grains, Pasta & Flour)						

*Less than 2% U.S. RDA

Sodium (mg)	Potassium (mg)	Protein (g)	Carbohy-drate (g)	Sugars (g)	Calcium (% U.S. RDA)	Iron (% U.S. RDA)	Vitamin A (% U.S. RDA)	Vitamin C (% U.S. RDA)
250	N.A.	3	18	N.A.	2	10	10	*
150	N.A.	2	15	N.A.	4	2	*	*
220	70	4	17	N.A.	4	*	*	*

∿ BREAKFAST CEREALS

∿ *Cereals are listed alphabetically by name; this category is the one for which listings are currently most complete.*

BREAKFAST CEREALS	Calories	Saturated fat (g)	Polyunsaturated fat (g)	Total fat (g)	Calories from fat	Cholesterol (mg)
All Bran (Kellogg), ⅓ oz (⅓ cup)	70	N.A.	N.A.	1	10	0
with extra fiber, 1 oz (½ cup)	50	0	0	0	0	0
Almond Delight (Ralston), 1 oz (¾ cup)	110	N.A.	N.A.	2	18	0
Alpha-Bits (Post), 1 oz (1 cup), all varieties	110	N.A.	N.A.	1	10	0
Apple Jacks (Kellogg), 1 oz (1 cup)	110	0	0	0	0	0
Apple Raisin Crisp (Kellogg), 1.3 oz (⅔ cup)	130	0	0	0	0	0
Basic 4 (General Mills), 1.3 oz (¾ cup)	130	N.A.	N.A.	2	18	0
Bigg Mixx (Kellogg), 1 oz (½ cup)	110	N.A.	N.A.	2	18	0
with raisins, 1.3 oz (½ cup)	140	N.A.	N.A.	2	18	0
Boo Berry (General Mills), 1 oz (1 cup)	110	N.A.	N.A.	1	10	0
Bran Buds (Kellogg), 1 oz (⅓ cup)	70	N.A.	N.A.	1	10	0
Bran Flakes (Kellogg), 1 oz (⅔ cup)	90	0	0	0	0	0
Bran Flakes (Post), 1 oz (⅔ cup)	90	0	0	0	0	0
Bran News (Ralston), 1 oz (¾ cup), all varieties	100	0	0	0	0	0
C.W. Post Hearty Granola, 1 oz (¼ cup)	130	N.A.	N.A.	4	35	0
Cap'n Crunch (Quaker), 1 oz (¾ cup)	120	<1	<1	2	18	N.A.
Cereal bars, Smart Start (Kellogg), 1 bar, all varieties	160	N.A.	N.A.	6	50	0
Cheerios (General Mills), 1 oz (1¼ cups)	110	N.A.	N.A.	2	18	0
flavored, 1 oz (¾ cup)	110	N.A.	N.A.	2	18	0

*Less than 2% U.S. RDA

Sodium (mg)	Potassium (mg)	Protein (g)	Carbohydrate (g)	Dietary fiber (g)	Sugars (g)	Calcium (% U.S. RDA)	Iron (% U.S. RDA)	Vitamin A (% U.S. RDA)	Vitamin C (% U.S. RDA)
260	320	4	22	10	5	2	25	15	25
140	330	4	22	14	0	2	25	15	25
200	N.A.	2	29	1	10	*	10	*	25
160	50	2	24	N.A.	12	*	15	25	*
125	30	2	26	1	14	*	25	15	25
230	115	2	32	3	11	*	10	15	*
230	110	3	28	2	8	20	25	25	25
190	55	2	24	1	8	*	25	15	*
190	110	2	31	2	14	*	25	15	*
210	45	1	24	N.A.	13	2	25	25	25
170	310	3	22	8	7	2	25	15	25
220	170	3	23	5	5	*	100	15	*
210	190	3	23	5	5	*	45	25	*
160	85	2	23	3	9	*	25	*	*
80	55	2	21	N.A.	N.A.	*	25	25	N.A.
240	40	1	24	0.8	12	*	25	*	*
150	75	2	25	1.2	10	2	10	15	*
290	105	4	20	2	1	4	45	25	25
220	80	3	23	1.5	10	2	25	25	25

~ BREAKFAST CEREALS	Calories	Saturated fat (g)	Polyunsaturated fat (g)	Total fat (g)	Calories from fat	Cholesterol (mg)
Chex (Ralston), 1 oz (½ to 1⅛ cups), all varieties	100	N.A.	N.A.	<1	N.A.	0
Chex Snack Mix (see Crackers, Chips, and Other Snacks)						
Clusters (General Mills), 1 oz (½ cup)	110	N.A.	N.A.	3	25	0
Cocoa Krispies (Kellogg), 1 oz (¾ cup)	110	0	0	0	0	0
Cocoa Pebbles (Post), 1 oz (⅞ cup)	110	N.A.	N.A.	1	10	0
Cocoa Puffs (General Mills), 1 oz (1 cup)	110	N.A.	N.A.	1	10	0
Common Sense Oat Bran (Kellogg), 1 oz (½ cup)	100	N.A.	N.A.	1	10	0
with raisins	120	0	0	0	0	0
Corn flake crumbs (Kellogg), 1 oz (¼ cup)	100	0	0	0	0	0
Corn Flakes (Kellogg), 1 oz (1 cup)	100	0	0	0	0	0
Corn Pops (Kellogg), 1 oz (1 cup)	110	0	0	0	0	0
Count Chocula (General Mills), 1 oz (1 cup)	110	N.A.	N.A.	1	10	0
Cracklin' Oat Bran (Kellogg), 1 oz (½ cup)	110	1	0	4	35	0
Cream of Rice (Nabisco), 1 oz (2½ tbsp uncooked)	100	0	0	0	0	N.A.
Cream of Wheat (Nabisco), 1 oz regular and instant (2½ tbsp uncooked)	100	0	0	0	0	0
Instant Mix & Eat, 1 packet original flavor	100	0	0	0	0	0
1 packet flavored	130	0	0	0	0	0
Quick, 1 oz (2½ tbsp uncooked)	100	0	0	0	0	0

*Less than 2% U.S. RDA
†Cooked without salt.

Sodium (mg)	Potassium (mg)	Protein (g)	Carbohy-drate (g)	Dietary fiber (g)	Sugars (g)	Calcium (% U.S. RDA)	Iron (% U.S. RDA)	Vitamin A (% U.S. RDA)	Vitamin C (% U.S. RDA)
230	70	2	24	N.A.	5	*	40	*	25
140	140	3	20	3	7	4	25	25	25
190	45	1	25	N.A.	11	*	10	15	25
160	45	1	25	N.A.	13	*	10	25	*
170	50	1	25	N.A.	14	*	25	*	25
270	115	4	22	3	5	*	25	15	*
250	170	4	29	3	10	2	25	15	*
290	35	2	24	N.A.	N.A.	*	10	*	25
290	35	2	24	1	2	*	10	15	25
90	20	1	26	N.A.	12	*	10	15	25
210	60	2	24	N.A.	13	2	25	25	25
150	160	3	20	4	7	*	10	15	25
0†	N.A.	2	23	N.A.	N.A.	*	6	*	*
0†	N.A.	3	22	1	<1	4	45	*	*
180	30	3	21	1	0	4	45	25	*
240	55	2	30	1	13	4	45	25	*
80	N.A.	3	22	1	<1	4	45	*	*

~ BREAKFAST CEREALS	Calories	Saturated fat (g)	Polyunsaturated fat (g)	Total fat (g)	Calories from fat	Cholesterol (mg)
Crispix (Kellogg), 1 oz (1 cup)	110	0	0	0	0	0
Crispy Rice (Ralston), 1 oz (1 cup)	110	0	0	0	0	0
Crispy Wheats 'n Raisins (General Mills), 1 oz (¾ cup)	100	N.A.	N.A.	1	10	0
Crunchy Rice Bran (Quaker), 1 oz (⅔ cup)	100	N.A.	N.A.	1	10	0
Farina, 1 cup cooked	120	0	0	<1	N.A.	0
Fiber One (General Mills), 1 oz (½ cup)	60	N.A.	N.A.	1	10	0
Froot Loops (Kellogg), 1 oz (1 cup)	110	N.A.	N.A.	1	10	0
Frosted Flakes (Kellogg), 1 oz (¾ cup)	110	0	0	0	0	0
Frosted Mini-Wheats (Kellogg), 1 oz (4 biscuits)	100	0	0	0	0	0
Frosted Wheat Squares (Nabisco), 1 oz (½ cup)	90	0	0	0	0	0
Fruit & Fibre (Post), 1.25 oz (⅔ cup)	120	N.A.	N.A.	3	25	0
Fruit Wheats (Nabisco), 1 oz (½ cup)	90	0	0	0	0	0
Fruitful Bran (Kellogg), 1.4 oz (⅔ cup)	120	N.A.	N.A.	1	10	0
Fruity Marshmallow Krispies (Kellogg), 1.3 oz (1¼ cups)	140	0	0	0	0	0
Fruity Pebbles (Post), 1 oz (⅞ cup)	110	N.A.	N.A.	1	10	0
Golden Grahams (General Mills), 1 oz (¾ cup)	110	N.A.	N.A.	1	10	0
Granola, Sun Country (Quaker), 1 oz (¼ cup), all varieties	120	1	1	5	45	0
Granola bars, 1 bar, all varieties	140	2	<1	6	50	0

*Less than 2% U.S. RDA
†Cooked without salt.

Sodium (mg)	Potassium (mg)	Protein (g)	Carbohy-drate (g)	Dietary fiber (g)	Sugars (g)	Calcium (% U.S. RDA)	Iron (% U.S. RDA)	Vitamin A (% U.S. RDA)	Vitamin C (% U.S. RDA)
220	30	2	25	N.A.	3	*	10	15	25
290	35	2	25	N.A.	3	*	10	25	25
140	120	2	23	2	10	4	25	25	*
250	120	2	22	2	6	*	45	*	*
0†	30	3	25	N.A.	N.A.	*	8	N.A.	N.A.
140	250	2	23	13	0	4	25	25	25
125	30	2	25	1	13	*	25	15	100
200	25	1	26	N.A.	11	*	10	15	25
0	80	3	24	3	6	*	10	*	*
15	90	2	23	3	5	*	10	15	*
170	210	3	27	5	10	*	35	30	*
15	90	2	23	3	5	*	10	15	*
220	230	3	31	5	13	*	25	15	*
210	20	2	32	N.A.	17	*	10	15	25
160	20	1	25	N.A.	12	*	10	25	*
280	55	1	24	N.A.	9	*	25	25	25
10	115	3	19	1.7	7	2	6	*	*
75	85	3	17	1.1	N.A.	2	4	*	*

～ BREAKFAST CEREALS	Calories	Saturated fat (g)	Polyunsaturated fat (g)	Total fat (g)	Calories from fat	Cholesterol (mg)
Grape-nuts (Post), 1 oz (¼ cup)	110	0	0	0	0	0
Grape-nuts Flakes (Post), 1 oz (⅞ cup)	100	N.A.	N.A.	1	10	0
Grits, corn, white or yellow, 1 cup cooked	150	<1	<1	<1	N.A.	0
Instant (Quaker), 1 pouch, all varieties	90	N.A.	N.A.	<1	N.A.	0
Quick (Quaker), 1 oz (3 tbsp uncooked)	100	0	0	0	0	N.A.
Heartwise (Kellogg), 1 oz (1 cup)	90	N.A.	N.A.	1	10	0
Honey Bunches of Oats (Post), 1 oz (⅔ cup), honey-roasted, with almonds	120	N.A.	N.A.	3	25	0
Honey Smacks (Kellogg), 1 oz (¾ cup)	110	N.A.	N.A.	1	10	0
Honeycomb (Post), 1 oz (1⅓ cups)	110	0	0	0	0	0
Just Right (Kellogg), 1 oz (⅔ cup), with fiber nuggets	100	N.A.	N.A.	1	10	0
with fruit and nuts, 1.3 oz (¾ cup)	140	N.A.	N.A.	1	10	0
Kaboom (General Mills), 1 oz (1 cup)	110	N.A.	N.A.	1	10	0
Kenmei Rice Bran (Kellogg), 1 oz (¾ cup)	110	N.A.	N.A.	1	10	0
with almond and raisin, 1.4 oz (¾ cup)	150	N.A.	N.A.	2	18	0
King Vitaman (Quaker), 1 oz (1¼ cups)	110	N.A.	N.A.	1	10	N.A.
Kix (General Mills), 1 oz (1½ cups)	110	N.A.	N.A.	1	10	0
Life (Quaker), 1 oz (⅔ cup)	100	N.A.	N.A.	2	18	N.A.
Lucky Charms (General Mills), 1 oz (1 cup)	110	N.A.	N.A.	1	10	0

*Less than 2% U.S. RDA
†Cooked without salt.

Sodium (mg)	Potassium (mg)	Protein (g)	Carbohy-drate (g)	Dietary fiber (g)	Sugars (g)	Calcium (% U.S. RDA)	Iron (% U.S. RDA)	Vitamin A (% U.S. RDA)	Vitamin C (% U.S. RDA)
170	90	3	23	2	3	*	45	25	*
160	85	3	23	3	5	*	45	25	*
0	55	4	31	N.A.	N.A.	*	10	*	N.A.
560	50	3	21	1.4	N.A.	*	45	*	*
0†	30	2	22	N.A.	N.A.	*	4	*	*
125	180	3	23	6	5	2	25	15	*
170	55	2	23	1	6	*	15	25	*
70	40	2	25	1	15	*	10	15	25
170	35	2	25	N.A.	11	*	15	25	*
200	70	2	24	2	5	*	100	15	*
190	120	3	30	2	9	*	100	15	*
290	60	2	23	N.A.	6	4	45	45	45
250	60	2	24	1	4	6	2	15	*
230	120	3	32	2	9	6	4	15	*
280	50	2	23	1.2	6	*	45	30	40
260	40	2	24	N.A.	3	4	45	25	25
190	170	5	19	2.5	5	8	45	*	*
180	70	2	24	N.A.	11	2	25	25	25

∿ BREAKFAST CEREALS	Calories	Saturated fat (g)	Polyunsaturated fat (g)	Total fat (g)	Calories from fat	Cholesterol (mg)
Maypo 30-second oatmeal, 1 oz (¼ cup uncooked)	100	N.A.	N.A.	1	10	0
Muesli (Ralston), 1.45 oz (½ cup), all varieties	150	N.A.	N.A.	3	25	0
Mueslix (Kellogg), 1.2 oz (½ cup)	130	N.A.	N.A.	3	25	0
with raisins, dates, almonds, 1.5 oz (⅔ cup)	160	N.A.	N.A.	2	18	0
Nature Valley 100% Natural (General Mills), 1 oz (⅓ cup), all varieties	130	N.A.	N.A.	5	45	0
Nut & Honey Crunch (Kellogg), 1 oz (⅔ cup)	110	N.A.	N.A.	1	10	0
Nut & Honey Crunch O's (Kellogg), 1 oz (⅔ cup)	110	N.A.	N.A.	2	18	0
Nutri-Grain (Kellogg), almond raisin, 1.4 oz (⅔ cup)	140	N.A.	N.A.	2	18	0
raisin bran, 1.4 oz (1 cup)	130	0	1	1	10	0
wheat, 1 oz (⅔ cup)	100	0	0	0	0	0
Oat Bran (Quaker), 1 oz (¾ cup)	100	<1	<1	2	18	0
Oat Bran (Nabisco), 1 oz (⅓ cup uncooked)	90	0	1	2	18	0
instant, 1 packet regular flavor	80	0	1	2	18	0
1 packet flavored	120	0	1	2	18	0
Oat Bran Flakes, 100% Organic (Health Valley), 1 oz (½ cup)	90	N.A.	N.A.	<1	N.A.	0
Oat Bran Options (Ralston), 1.45 oz (1 cup)	130	N.A.	N.A.	1	10	0
Oat Bran O's (Health Valley), 1 oz (½ cup)	90	N.A.	N.A.	<1	N.A.	0
Oat Flakes (Post), 1 oz (⅔ cup)	110	N.A.	N.A.	1	10	0

*Less than 2% U.S. RDA
†Cooked without salt.

Sodium (mg)	Potassium (mg)	Protein (g)	Carbohy-drate (g)	Dietary fiber (g)	Sugars (g)	Calcium (% U.S. RDA)	Iron (% U.S. RDA)	Vitamin A (% U.S. RDA)	Vitamin C (% U.S. RDA)
0†	95	4	19	N.A.	3	8	45	30	30
95	180	4	31	3	11	*	20	25	*
170	115	3	25	2	7	2	25	15	*
150	160	3	33	3	13	4	25	4	*
85	80	2	20	1	6	*	4	*	*
200	40	2	24	N.A.	9	*	10	15	25
190	70	2	22	1	12	2	10	15	25
220	130	3	31	3	7	*	4	*	*
200	250	4	31	5	9	20	10	*	*
170	90	3	24	3	2	*	4	*	25
125	135	5	20	3	4	*	30	20	*
0†	160	4	20	5	0	2	25	25	*
0	140	4	20	5	0	2	25	25	*
160	160	1	28	5	10	2	25	25	*
0	105	3	20	3.7	N.A.	*	6	*	*
150	190	4	32	3	12	2	45	10	*
0	105	3	20	3.7	N.A.	*	6	*	*
130	135	4	21	2	6	2	45	25	*

~ BREAKFAST CEREALS	Calories	Saturated fat (g)	Polyunsat- urated fat (g)	Total fat (g)	Calories from fat	Choles- terol (mg)
Oat Squares (Quaker), 1 oz (½ cup)	100	N.A.	N.A.	2	18	N.A.
Oatbake (Kellogg), 1 oz (⅓ cup), all varieties	110	1	1	3	25	0
Oatmeal, Old Fashioned Quaker, regular and quick, 1 oz (⅓ cup uncooked)	100	N.A.	N.A.	2	18	0
instant, 1 packet, all varieties	120	N.A.	N.A.	2	18	0
Oatmeal Crisp (General Mills), 1 oz (1 cup)	110	N.A.	N.A.	2	18	0
Oatmeal Raisin Crisp (General Mills), 1 oz (½ cup)	110	N.A.	N.A.	2	18	0
Oatmeal Swirlers (General Mills), 1 packet, all varieties	160	N.A.	N.A.	2	18	0
Oh!s (Quaker), 1 oz (⅔ to 1 cup), all varieties	120	2	<1	2	18	0
100% Bran (Nabisco), 1 oz (½ cup)	70	N.A.	N.A.	2	18	N.A.
Product 19 (Kellogg), 1 oz (1 cup)	100	0	0	0	0	0
Puffed Rice (Quaker), ½ oz (1 heaping cup)	50	0	0	0	0	0
Puffed Wheat (Quaker), ½ oz (1 heaping cup)	50	0	0	0	0	0
Raisin Bran (Kellogg), 1.4 oz (¾ cup)	120	N.A.	N.A.	1	10	0
Raisin Bran (Post), 1.4 oz (⅔ cup)	120	N.A.	N.A.	1	10	0
Raisin Nut Bran (General Mills), 1 oz (½ cup)	110	N.A.	N.A.	3	25	0
Raisin Oat Bran (General Mills), 1.5 oz (¾ cup)	150	N.A.	N.A.	2	18	0
Ralston High Fiber Cereal, 1 oz (⅓ cup uncooked)	90	N.A.	N.A.	1	10	0

*Less than 2% U.S. RDA
†Cooked without salt.

Sodium (mg)	Potassium (mg)	Protein (g)	Carbohy-drate (g)	Dietary fiber (g)	Sugars (g)	Calcium (% U.S. RDA)	Iron (% U.S. RDA)	Vitamin A (% U.S. RDA)	Vitamin C (% U.S. RDA)
160	100	4	21	2.4	5	2	35	30	*
190	100	2	21	2	8	*	25	15	25
0†	100	5	18	2.7	N.A.	*	6	*	*
210	100	4	25	2.5	N.A.	20	45	25	*
180	80	2	22	1	6	4	25	25	25
140	100	2	21	1	8	6	25	25	*
110	85	3	34	2	19	6	25	25	25
170	45	2	23	0.9	9	*	30	15	10
190	N.A.	3	21	10	6	2	15	*	45
320	45	3	24	1	3	*	100	15	100
0	20	1	13	0.2	0	*	2	*	*
0	55	2	11	1	0	*	2	*	*
230	250	3	30	5	12	2	100	15	*
200	260	3	31	6	14	*	35	35	*
140	140	3	20	2.5	8	4	25	25	*
130	200	4	31	3	14	2	25	25	*
5†	105	3	21	4	0	*	4	*	*

～ BREAKFAST CEREALS	Calories	Saturated fat (g)	Polyunsaturated fat (g)	Total fat (g)	Calories from fat	Cholesterol (mg)
Rice Bran, Crunchy (Quaker), 1 oz (⅔ cup)	100	N.A.	N.A.	1	10	0
Rice Bran, Honey Crunch (Quaker), 1 oz (¼ cup)	100	N.A.	N.A.	5	45	0
Rice Bran Options (Ralston), 1.12 oz (1 cup)	120	N.A.	N.A.	2	18	0
Rice Krispies (Kellogg), 1 oz (1 cup)	110	0	0	0	0	0
Shredded Wheat (Quaker), 1.4 oz (2 biscuits)	130	N.A.	N.A.	1	10	N.A.
Shredded Wheat 'n Bran (Nabisco), 1 oz (⅔ cup)	90	N.A.	N.A.	<1	N.A.	0
Shredded Wheat Squares (Kellogg), 1 oz (½ cup)	90	0	0	0	0	0
Special K (Kellogg), 1 oz (1 cup)	110	0	0	0	0	0
Sprouts with Raisins, 100% Organic (Health Valley), 1 oz (¼ cup)	90	N.A.	N.A.	<1	N.A.	0
Sunflakes Multi-Grain (Ralston), 1 oz (1 cup)	100	N.A.	N.A.	1	10	0
Super Golden Crisp (Post), 1 oz (⅞ cup)	100	0	0	0	0	0
Teddy Grahams Breakfast Bears (Nabisco), 1 oz (⅓ cup)	120	<1	<1	3	25	0
Toasted Wheat Bran (Kretschmer), 1 oz (¼ cup)	40	N.A.	N.A.	2	18	0
Total (General Mills), 1 oz (1 cup)	100	N.A.	N.A.	1	10	0
Total Corn Flakes (General Mills), 1 oz (1 cup)	110	N.A.	N.A.	1	10	0
Total Oatmeal (General Mills)						
Instant, 1 packet, regular	110	N.A.	N.A.	2	18	0
flavored	160	N.A.	N.A.	2	18	0
Quick, 1 packet	90	N.A.	N.A.	2	18	0

*Less than 2% U.S. RDA

Sodium (mg)	Potassium (mg)	Protein (g)	Carbohy-drate (g)	Dietary fiber (g)	Sugars (g)	Calcium (% U.S. RDA)	Iron (% U.S. RDA)	Vitamin A (% U.S. RDA)	Vitamin C (% U.S. RDA)
250	120	2	22	2	6	*	45	*	*
5	340	3	15	5	6	2	20	2	*
120	140	3	24	3	7	2	45	10	25
290	35	2	25	0	3	*	10	15	25
0	150	4	32	4	0	2	6	*	*
0	140	3	23	4	<1	*	8	*	*
0	110	2	23	2	6	*	45	*	*
230	55	6	20	N.A.	3	*	25	15	25
0	130	4	16	4.7	N.A.	*	8	2	*
240	N.A.	2	24	3	0	*	10	25	25
45	40	2	26	N.A.	15	*	10	25	*
135	40	2	22	1	7	*	25	25	*
0	460	4	16	14.1	N.A.	2	20	*	*
140	110	3	22	3	3	20	100	100	100
280	35	2	24	N.A.	2	20	100	100	100
220	110	4	22	3	3	20	100	100	100
130	140	4	35	3	16	20	100	100	100
0	100	4	18	3	0	20	100	100	100

~ BREAKFAST CEREALS	Calories	Saturated fat (g)	Polyunsaturated fat (g)	Total fat (g)	Calories from fat	Cholesterol (mg)
Total Raisin Bran (General Mills), 1.5 oz (1 cup)	140	N.A.	N.A.	1	10	0
Total Whole Wheat (General Mills), 1 oz (1 cup)	100	N.A.	N.A.	1	10	0
Triples (General Mills), 1 oz (¾ cup)	110	N.A.	N.A.	1	10	0
Trix (General Mills), 1 oz (1 cup)	110	N.A.	N.A.	1	10	0
Wheat Germ (Kretschmer), 1 oz (3 tbsp)	100	1	2	3	25	0
Wheat Hearts (General Mills), 1 oz (3⅓ tbsp uncooked)	110	N.A.	N.A.	1	10	0
Wheatena Toasted Wheat Cereal, 1 oz (¼ cup uncooked)	100	N.A.	N.A.	1	10	0
Wheaties (General Mills), 1 oz (1 cup)	100	N.A.	N.A.	1	10	0

*Less than 2% U.S. RDA
†Cooked without salt.

Sodium (mg)	Potassium (mg)	Protein (g)	Carbohy-drate (g)	Dietary fiber (g)	Sugars (g)	Calcium (% U.S. RDA)	Iron (% U.S. RDA)	Vitamin A (% U.S. RDA)	Vitamin C (% U.S. RDA)
190	220	3	33	4	14	20	100	100	*
200	110	3	23	3	3	20	100	100	100
250	35	2	24	N.A.	3	2	25	25	25
140	25	1	25	N.A.	12	*	25	25	25
0	300	9	12	3.3	3	*	10	*	*
0†	105	4	21	N.A.	1	*	45	*	*
0†	100	3	21	4	N.A.	*	6	*	*
200	110	3	23	3	3	6	45	25	25

∽ CANDY

∽ SUGARS

∽ SYRUPS

∽ & TOPPINGS

∽ *Candies are listed first, alphabetically by name. Sugar listings are included where available; fiber is not listed, since these products contain minimal amounts.*

~ CANDY

	Calories	Saturated fat (g)	Polyunsat-urated fat (g)	Total fat (g)	Calories from fat	Choles-terol (mg)
After Eight Chocolate Wafer Thin Mints (Nestlé), 1 mint	35	N.A.	N.A.	1	10	N.A.
Almond Joy Bar (Hershey), 1.76 oz	250	N.A.	N.A.	14	130	0
Alpine White Bar with Al-monds (Nestlé), 1.25 oz	200	N.A.	N.A.	13	120	N.A.
Andes Crème de Menthe Day-dreams, 1 oz (6 pieces)	150	N.A.	N.A.	9	80	N.A.
Baby Ruth Bar (Nestlé), 2.2 oz	300	6	2	13	120	0
Bar None (Hershey), 1.5 oz	240	N.A.	N.A.	14	130	10
Berry Bears (General Mills), 1 pouch, all flavors	100	N.A.	N.A.	<1	N.A.	N.A.
Bit-O-Honey Bar (Nestlé), 1.7 oz	200	N.A.	N.A.	4	35	N.A.
Bounty Bars (Mars), 1 bar (1.05 oz), dark, milk	150	N.A.	N.A.	8	70	N.A.
Butterfinger (Nestlé), 2.1 oz bar	280	5	2	12	110	0
Butterscotch disks (Brach's), 1 oz	110	0	0	0	0	N.A.
Butterscotch-flavored morsels (Nestlé), 1 oz	150	N.A.	N.A.	8	70	N.A.
Cadbury's Dairy Milk Choco-late, 1 oz	150	N.A.	N.A.	8	70	N.A.
Caramello Bar (Hershey), 1.6 oz	220	N.A.	N.A.	11	100	10
Caramels (Brach's milk maid), 1 oz	110	N.A.	N.A.	2	18	N.A.
Caroby Milk Bar (Natural Touch), Worthington Foods, 1 oz (⅓ of bar)	150	N.A.	N.A.	9	80	N.A.
Chunky Bar (Nestlé), 1.4 oz	210	N.A.	N.A.	12	110	N.A.
Circus Peanuts (Brach's), 1 oz	100	0	0	0	0	N.A.
5th Avenue Bar (Hershey), 2.1 oz	290	N.A.	N.A.	13	120	5
Fruit Roll-Ups (General Mills), ½-oz roll, all flavors	50	N.A.	N.A.	<1	N.A.	N.A.

*Less than 2% U.S. RDA

Sodium (mg)	Potassium (mg)	Protein (g)	Carbohy-drate (g)	Sugars (g)	Calcium (% U.S. RDA)	Iron (% U.S. RDA)	Vitamin A (% U.S. RDA)	Vitamin C (% U.S. RDA)
0	15	0	6	N.A.	*	*	*	*
70	N.A.	3	28	22	2	2	*	*
30	140	4	18	N.A.	10	*	*	*
15	N.A.	2	16	N.A.	4	6	*	*
130	N.A.	5	40	N.A.	2	4	*	*
50	N.A.	4	23	19	6	2	*	*
20	35	<1	22	N.A.	*	*	*	*
125	N.A.	1	39	N.A.	2	*	*	*
50	N.A.	1	18	N.A.	*	2	*	*
105	N.A.	4	41	N.A.	2	4	*	*
220	N.A.	0	27	N.A.	*	*	*	*
25	55	1	19	N.A.	*	*	*	*
45	N.A.	2	17	N.A.	6	4	*	*
60	N.A.	3	28	23	8	2	*	*
70	N.A.	1	23	N.A.	*	*	*	*
55	N.A.	4	13	N.A.	15	2	*	*
20	N.A.	4	22	N.A.	6	4	*	*
10	N.A.	0	26	N.A.	*	*	*	*
140	N.A.	5	39	31	4	*	*	*
40	25	<1	12	N.A.	*	*	*	*

	Calories	Saturated fat (g)	Polyunsaturated fat (g)	Total fat (g)	Calories from fat	Cholesterol (mg)
Fruit Wrinkles (General Mills), 1 pouch, all flavors	100	N.A.	N.A.	1	10	N.A.
Garfield & Friends (General Mills), 1 pouch, 1-2 punch, very strawberry	100	N.A.	N.A.	2	18	N.A.
½-oz roll, fruit party, wild blue	50	N.A.	N.A.	<1	N.A.	N.A.
Golden Almond Chocolate Bar (Hershey), ½ bar (1.6 oz)	260	N.A.	N.A.	17	150	5
Golden III Chocolate Bar (Hershey), ½ bar (1.6 oz)	250	N.A.	N.A.	15	140	10
Goobers Chocolate Covered Peanuts (Nestlé), 1⅜ oz	220	N.A.	N.A.	13	120	N.A.
Hershey's Kisses, 9 pieces (1.5 oz)	220	N.A.	N.A.	13	120	10
with almonds, 9 pieces (1.5 oz)	240	N.A.	N.A.	15	N.A.	N.A.
Hershey's Milk Chocolate Bar, 1.55 oz	240	N.A.	N.A.	14	130	10
with almonds, 1.45 oz	230	N.A.	N.A.	14	130	15
Holidays (Mars), 1 oz	140	N.A.	N.A.	6	50	N.A.
Jellybeans (Brach's), 1 oz	100	0	0	0	0	N.A.
Kit Kat Bar (Hershey), 1.6 oz	250	N.A.	N.A.	13	120	10
Krackel Bar (Hershey), 1.55 oz	230	N.A.	N.A.	13	120	10
Lemon Drops (Brach's), 1 oz	110	0	0	0	0	N.A.
Life Savers, 1 piece, all flavors, roll candy, Breath Savers mints	8	0	0	0	0	N.A.
Lollipops (Life Savers), 1	45	0	0	0	0	N.A.
M&M's, plain, 1.69-oz pkg	250	N.A.	N.A.	12	110	N.A.
peanut, 1.74-oz pkg	250	N.A.	N.A.	13	120	N.A.
Mars Bar (Mars), 1.76 oz	240	N.A.	N.A.	11	100	N.A.
Marshmallows (Campfire), 2 large or 24 mini	40	0	0	0	0	N.A.
Milky Way Bar (Mars), 2.15 oz	280	N.A.	N.A.	11	100	N.A.

*Less than 2% U.S. RDA

Sodium (mg)	Potassium (mg)	Protein (g)	Carbohy-drate (g)	Sugars (g)	Calcium (% U.S. RDA)	Iron (% U.S. RDA)	Vitamin A (% U.S. RDA)	Vitamin C (% U.S. RDA)
55	45	<1	22	N.A.	*	*	*	*
65	55	<1	21	N.A.	*	*	*	*
30	35	<1	12	N.A.	*	*	*	*
35	N.A.	5	20	17	10	2	*	*
40	N.A.	3	26	23	10	*	*	*
15	N.A.	6	19	N.A.	4	2	*	*
35	N.A.	3	23	22	8	2	*	*
40	N.A.	5	21	N.A.	10	4	*	*
40	N.A.	4	25	23	8	*	*	*
55	N.A.	5	20	18	10	4	*	*
40	N.A.	2	19	N.A.	4	2	*	*
10	N.A.	0	26	17	*	*	*	*
60	N.A.	3	29	23	10	2	*	*
80	N.A.	3	27	22	8	*	*	*
5	N.A.	0	27	N.A.	*	*	*	*
5	0	0	2	N.A.	*	*	*	*
10	0	0	11	N.A.	*	*	*	*
70	N.A.	3	34	N.A.	8	4	*	*
55	N.A.	6	29	N.A.	6	2	*	*
85	N.A.	4	30	N.A.	8	2	*	*
10	0	0	20	N.A.	*	*	*	*
150	N.A.	3	42	N.A.	6	2	*	*

	Calories	Saturated fat (g)	Polyunsaturated fat (g)	Total fat (g)	Calories from fat	Cholesterol (mg)
dark bar, 1.76 oz	220	N.A.	N.A.	8	70	N.A.
Mints (Brach's), 1 oz, mint coolers, peppermint starlight mints (Kentucky mints have 0 mg sodium)	110	0	0	0	0	N.A.
Mr. Goodbar (Hershey), 1.75 oz	290	N.A.	N.A.	19	170	15
Mounds Bar (Hershey), 1.9 oz	260	N.A.	N.A.	14	130	0
Munch Bar (Mars), 1.42 oz	220	N.A.	N.A.	14	130	N.A.
Nestlé Crunch, 1 bar (1.4 oz)	210	N.A.	N.A.	10	90	N.A.
Nestlé Milk Chocolate Bar (1.45 oz)	220	N.A.	N.A.	13	120	N.A.
with almonds (1.45 oz)	230	N.A.	N.A.	14	130	N.A.
Oh Henry! Bar (Nestlé), 2 oz	280	N.A.	N.A.	14	130	N.A.
100 Grand Bar (Nestlé), 1.5 oz	200	N.A.	N.A.	8	70	N.A.
Orangettes jelly candy (Brach's), 1 oz	100	0	0	0	0	N.A.
PB Max Snack (Mars), 1.48 oz	240	N.A.	N.A.	16	140	N.A.
Peanut Bar (Planters), 1.6 oz, regular	230	2	4	11	100	0
honey-roasted	230	2	4	13	120	0
sweet 'n crunchy	250	2	4	15	140	0
Peanut Candy, Old Fashioned (Planters), 1 oz	140	1	3	9	80	0
Pearson Nips & Parfaits, all flavors, 1 oz	120	N.A.	N.A.	3	25	N.A.
Raisinets (Nestlé), 1⅜-oz pkg	180	N.A.	N.A.	6	35	N.A.
Reese's Peanut Butter Cup (Hershey), 1.8 oz	280	N.A.	N.A.	17	150	10
Reese's Peanut Butter flavored chips, ¼ cup (1.5 oz)	230	N.A.	N.A.	13	120	5
Reese's Pieces (Hershey), 8 pieces	260	N.A.	N.A.	11	100	5
Rolo Caramels (Hershey), 8 pieces	270	N.A.	N.A.	12	110	15

*Less than 2% U.S. RDA

Sodium (mg)	Potassium (mg)	Protein (g)	Carbohydrate (g)	Sugars (g)	Calcium (% U.S. RDA)	Iron (% U.S. RDA)	Vitamin A (% U.S. RDA)	Vitamin C (% U.S. RDA)
115	N.A.	1	36	N.A.	2	2	*	*
15	N.A.	0	27	N.A.	*	*	*	*
20	N.A.	7	23	21	6	2	*	*
85	N.A.	2	31	23	*	4	*	*
110	N.A.	6	19	N.A.	2	2	*	*
35	85	3	26	N.A.	6	*	*	*
25	N.A.	3	25	N.A.	6	*	*	*
25	N.A.	4	22	N.A.	8	2	*	*
85	N.A.	6	32	N.A.	4	*	*	*
55	N.A.	2	31	N.A.	6	*	*	*
20	N.A.	0	24	N.A.	*	*	*	*
160	N.A.	5	20	N.A.	2	2	*	*
70	180	8	25	N.A.	*	2	*	*
150	170	6	25	N.A.	*	4	*	*
110	200	7	21	N.A.	*	4	*	*
70	130	4	13	N.A.	*	*	*	*
70	70	1	23	N.A.	2	*	*	*
10	150	2	28	N.A.	4	2	*	*
180	N.A.	6	26	24	2	2	*	*
90	N.A.	7	19	N.A.	6	4	*	*
90	N.A.	8	32	30	2	2	*	*
110	N.A.	3	37	33	6	*	*	*

~ CANDY/ SUGARS, SYRUPS & TOPPINGS	Calories	Saturated fat (g)	Polyunsat- urated fat (g)	Total fat (g)	Calories from fat	Choles- terol (mg)
Shark Bites (General Mills), 1 pouch, all flavors	100	N.A.	N.A.	<1	N.A.	N.A.
Skittles (Mars), 2.3 oz	270	N.A.	N.A.	3	25	N.A.
Skor Toffee Bar (Hershey), 1.4 oz	220	N.A.	N.A.	14	130	25
Snickers Bar (Mars), 2.07 oz	280	N.A.	N.A.	14	130	N.A.
peanut butter, 1.76 oz	280	N.A.	N.A.	18	160	N.A.
Sno-Caps Chocolate Nonpa- reils (Nestlé), 1 oz	140	N.A.	N.A.	5	45	N.A.
Solitaires Chocolate with Al- monds (Hershey), ½ bag (1.6 oz)	260	N.A.	N.A.	17	150	5
Sour balls (Brach's), 1 oz	110	0	0	0	0	N.A.
Spearmint leaves (Brach's), 1 oz	100	0	0	0	0	N.A.
Special Dark Bar (Hershey), 1.45 oz	220	N.A.	N.A.	12	110	0
Starburst Fruit Chews (Mars), 2.07 oz	240	N.A.	N.A.	5	45	N.A.
Symphony almond/butterchips (Hershey), 1.4 oz	220	N.A.	N.A.	14	130	N.A.
milk chocolate, 1.4 oz	220	N.A.	N.A.	13	120	10
3 Musketeers Bar (Mars), 2.13 oz	260	N.A.	N.A.	8	70	N.A.
Thunder Jets (General Mills), 1 pouch, all flavors	100	N.A.	N.A.	1	10	N.A.
Turtles Milk Chocolate Pecan Caramel, 1 piece (0.6 oz)	90	N.A.	N.A.	5	45	N.A.
Whatchamacallit Bar (Her- shey), 1.8 oz	260	N.A.	N.A.	13	120	10
Y&S Bites, Nibs, Twizzlers (Hershey), 1 oz	100	N.A.	N.A.	1	10	0
York Peppermint Patty (Her- shey), 1.5 oz	180	N.A.	N.A.	4	35	0
Apple butter, Bama, 2 tsp	25	0	0	0	0	N.A.
Chocolate						

*Less than 2% U.S. RDA

Sodium (mg)	Potassium (mg)	Protein (g)	Carbohy-drate (g)	Sugars (g)	Calcium (% U.S. RDA)	Iron (% U.S. RDA)	Vitamin A (% U.S. RDA)	Vitamin C (% U.S. RDA)
20	35	<1	22	N.A.	*	*	*	*
35	N.A.	0	60	N.A.	*	*	*	50
125	N.A.	2	22	20	2	*	*	*
160	N.A.	6	35	N.A.	6	2	*	*
135	N.A.	6	23	N.A.	4	2	*	*
0	75	1	21	N.A.	*	2	*	*
25	N.A.	6	20	17	10	2	*	*
15	N.A.	0	27	N.A.	*	*	*	*
10	N.A.	0	24	N.A.	*	*	*	*
5	N.A.	3	25	21	*	4	*	*
30	N.A.	0	48	N.A.	*	*	*	50
40	N.A.	4	20	18	8	2	*	*
35	N.A.	3	22	20	10	*	*	*
120	N.A.	2	46	N.A.	4	2	*	*
30	25	<1	22	N.A.	*	*	*	*
15	50	1	10	N.A.	2	*	*	*
130	N.A.	5	30	23	6	*	*	*
90	N.A.	1	23	12	*	*	*	*
20	N.A.	1	34	26	*	2	*	*
5	10	0	6	N.A.	*	*	*	*

~ SUGARS, SYRUPS & TOPPINGS	Calories	Saturated fat (g)	Polyunsaturated fat (g)	Total fat (g)	Calories from fat	Cholesterol (mg)
milk chocolate chips, ¼ cup (1.5 oz)	220	N.A.	N.A.	13	120	9
semisweet real chocolate chips, ¼ cup (1.5 oz)	210	N.A.	N.A.	12	110	0
chocolate flavored, ¼ cup (1.5 oz)	200	N.A.	N.A.	9	80	0
sweet German's bar, 1 oz	140	N.A.	N.A.	10	90	0
unsweetened bar, 1 oz	170	N.A.	N.A.	16	140	0
Chocolate Fudge Topping, Hershey's, 2 tbsp (1 oz)	100	N.A.	N.A.	4	35	5
Chocolate Syrup, Hershey's, 2 tbsp (1 oz)	80	N.A.	N.A.	1	10	0
Cocoa, dry, Hershey's, ⅓ cup	120	N.A.	N.A.	4	35	0
Corn syrup, 1 tbsp	60	0	0	0	0	N.A.
Dairy toppings (see Dairy Products & Eggs)						
Gum, chewing						
bubble gum, Bubble Yum	25	0	0	0	0	N.A.
sugarless	20	0	0	0	0	N.A.
regular, 1 piece	10	0	0	0	0	N.A.
sugarless	8	0	0	0	0	N.A.
Honey, 1 tbsp	60	0	0	0	0	N.A.
Jelly, jam, preserves, 2 tsp	30	0	0	0	0	N.A.
low calorie, Smucker's, 1 tsp	8	0	0	0	0	N.A.
Molasses, medium, 1 tbsp	45	0	0	0	0	N.A.
Pancake syrup, 2 tbsp	110	0	0	0	0	0
lite	50	N.A.	N.A.	<1	N.A.	0
Sugar						
brown, 1 cup loosely packed	540	0	0	0	0	N.A.
white, granulated, 1 tbsp	45	0	0	0	0	N.A.
1 cup	770	0	0	0	0	N.A.
white, powdered, 1 cup	460	0	0	0	0	N.A.
Sugar substitute, 1 serving	2	0	0	0	0	N.A.

Sodium (mg)	Potassium (mg)	Protein (g)	Carbohy-drate (g)	Sugars (g)	Calcium (% U.S. RDA)	Iron (% U.S. RDA)	Vitamin A (% U.S. RDA)	Vitamin C (% U.S. RDA)
55	140	3	26	25	8	*	*	*
0	135	2	27	24	*	8	*	*
30	220	2	30	N.A.	6	4	*	*
0	80	1	17	14	*	4	*	*
0	250	4	8	N.A.	2	10	*	*
30	N.A.	1	14	N.A.	2	2	*	*
20	N.A.	1	17	25	*	2	*	*
10	N.A.	7	13	N.A.	4	25	*	*
15	0	0	15	9	*	4	*	*
0	0	0	7	N.A.	*	*	*	*
0	0	0	5	N.A.	*	*	*	*
0	0	0	2	N.A.	*	*	*	*
0	0	0	2	N.A.	*	*	*	*
0	10	<1	17	17	*	*	*	*
5	10	0	8	N.A.	*	*	*	*
0	N.A.	0	2	N.A.	N.A.	N.A.	N.A.	N.A.
5	210	0	12	12	6	8	N.A.	N.A.
35	0	0	27	21	*	*	*	*
80	0	<1	13	15	*	*	*	*
45	500	0	140	140	10	30	*	*
0	0	0	12	12	*	*	*	*
0	5	0	199	199	*	*	*	*
0	0	0	119	119	*	*	*	*
1	0	0	<1	N.A.	*	*	*	*

∾ CONDIMENTS:

∾ Sauces

∾ Gravies

∾ & Seasonings

∾ Values for sugar and fiber content are not readily available and so are not included here. Baking powder and soda are also listed under Flours in "Grains, Pasta & Flour" for ease in calculating recipes. Salad dressings are listed in "Fats, Oils, Margarines & Salad Dressings" and also in the Salad Bar section of "Fast Foods."

	Calories	Saturated fat (g)	Polyunsaturated fat (g)	Total fat (g)	Calories from fat	Cholesterol (mg)
Baking powder, 1 tsp	4	0	0	0	0	0
low sodium, 1 tsp	8	0	0	0	0	N.A.
Baking soda, 1 tsp	N.A.	N.A.	N.A.	N.A.	N.A.	N.A.
Barbecue sauce						
Heinz, 1 tbsp, all varieties	20	0	0	0	0	N.A.
Hunt, 1 tbsp, all varieties	20	N.A.	N.A.	<1	N.A.	0
Bean dip						
Old El Paso, chili, 2 tbsp	16	N.A.	N.A.	<1	N.A.	N.A.
Wise, jalapeño flavor, 2 tbsp	25	0	0	0	0	N.A.
Cheese sauce (see Dairy Products & Eggs)						
Chili sauce						
El Molino, mild green, 2 tbsp	10	0	0	0	0	N.A.
Heinz, 1 tbsp	18	0	0	0	0	N.A.
Chilies, green, Old El Paso, 2 tbsp chopped	8	N.A.	N.A.	<1	N.A.	N.A.
Cocoa, dry (see Candy, Sugars, Syrups & Toppings)						
Cocktail sauce, seafood, Heinz, 1 tbsp	20	N.A.	N.A.	N.A.	N.A.	N.A.
Cream of tartar, 1 tbsp	8	0	0	0	0	N.A.
Enchilada sauce						
green, Old El Paso, 2 tbsp	12	0	0	0	0	0
hot, El Molino, 2 tbsp	16	N.A.	N.A.	1	10	N.A.
mild, El Molino, 2 tbsp	12	N.A.	N.A.	<1	N.A.	0
Fajita marinade, Old El Paso, ⅛ jar	14	0	0	0	0	0
Flavor enhancer, Ac'cent, ½ tsp	6	0	0	0	0	0
Gravy						
canned, 1 cup, au jus	40	<1	0	<1	N.A.	1
beef, 1 cup	120	3	<1	6	50	7
chicken, 1 cup	190	3	4	14	130	5

*Less than 2% U.S. RDA

Sodium (mg)	Potassium (mg)	Protein (g)	Carbohy-drate (g)	Calcium (% U.S. RDA)	Iron (% U.S. RDA)	Vitamin A (% U.S. RDA)	Vitamin C (% U.S. RDA)
430	0	<1	0	25	*	*	*
0	N.A.	0	2	*	*	*	*
1100	N.A.	N.A.	N.A.	N.A.	N.A.	N.A.	N.A.
220	N.A.	0	5	*	*	N.A.	N.A.
150	40	<1	5	*	*	*	4
100	50	0	3	*	*	*	*
100	105	1	5	*	2	*	*
210	60	0	2	*	*	8	*
190	N.A.	0	4	N.A.	N.A.	N.A.	N.A.
70	N.A.	<1	2	4	2	*	20
160	N.A.	N.A.	N.A.	N.A.	N.A.	N.A.	N.A.
690	360	2	0	*	*	*	*
200	20	<1	3	*	*	*	*
100	45	0	2	*	2	20	*
125	N.A.	<1	2	*	4	*	*
450	25	0	3	*	*	*	*
300	0	0	0	*	*	*	*
N.A.	N.A.	3	6	*	10	*	4
115	190	9	11	*	10	*	*
1380	260	5	13	4	8	20	*

~ CONDIMENTS

	Calories	Saturated fat (g)	Polyunsaturated fat (g)	Total fat (g)	Calories from fat	Cholesterol (mg)
mushroom, 1 cup	120	1	2	7	60	0
pork, Franco American, 1 cup	160	N.A.	N.A.	12	110	N.A.
turkey, 1 cup	120	2	1	5	45	5
dehydrated, prepared with water, 1 cup, chicken	80	<1	<1	2	18	3
mushroom, 1 cup	70	<1	0	<1	N.A.	1
onion, 1 cup	80	<1	0	<1	N.A.	1
Gravy, Brown seasoning, La Choy, ½ tsp	16	N.A.	N.A.	<1	N.A.	0
Heinz 57 Sauce, 1 tbsp	16	0	0	0	0	N.A.
Horseradish, prepared, 1 tbsp	6	0	0	0	N.A.	N.A.
Horseradish sauce, Heinz, 1 tbsp	75	N.A.	N.A.	7	60	N.A.
Ketchup						
Heinz, 1 tbsp	18	0	0	0	0	N.A.
lite, 1 tbsp	8	0	0	0	0	N.A.
low-sodium lite, 1 tbsp	8	0	0	0	0	N.A.
Hunt, 1 tbsp	16	N.A.	N.A.	<1	N.A.	0
no salt added, 1 tbsp	20	N.A.	N.A.	<1	N.A.	0
Weight Watchers, 2 tsp	8	0	0	0	0	N.A.
Lobster sauce, Progresso, ½ cup	120	1	3	8	70	10
Mexican seasoning mixes, Old El Paso						
burrito, ⅛ pkg	18	0	0	0	N.A.	0
chili, ⅕ pkg	20	N.A.	N.A.	1	10	0
enchilada, 1/18 pkg	6	0	0	0	N.A.	0
guacamole, ⅐ pkg	8	0	0	0	N.A.	0
taco, 1/12 pkg	8	N.A.	N.A.	<1	N.A.	0
Mrs. Dash seasoning, 1 tsp	12	0	0	0	0	N.A.
steak sauce, 1 tbsp	18	0	0	0	0	N.A.
Molly McButter, ½ tsp	4	0	0	0	0	0

*Less than 2% U.S. RDA

Sodium (mg)	Potassium (mg)	Protein (g)	Carbohy-drate (g)	Calcium (% U.S. RDA)	Iron (% U.S. RDA)	Vitamin A (% U.S. RDA)	Vitamin C (% U.S. RDA)
1360	250	3	13	*	10	*	*
1400	N.A.	0	12	N.A.	N.A.	N.A.	N.A.
N.A.	N.A.	6	12	*	10	*	*
1130	N.A.	3	14	4	N.A.	N.A.	N.A.
1400	N.A.	2	14	4	N.A.	N.A.	N.A.
1040	N.A.	2	17	6	N.A.	N.A.	N.A.
15	0	<1	4	*	*	*	*
270	N.A.	0	3	N.A.	N.A.	N.A.	N.A.
15	45	<1	1	*	*	N.A.	N.A.
115	N.A.	<1	2	N.A.	N.A.	N.A.	N.A.
180	N.A.	0	4	*	*	N.A.	N.A.
110	N.A.	0	2	*	*	N.A.	N.A.
90	N.A.	0	2	*	*	N.A.	N.A.
160	50	<1	4	*	*	*	4
0	60	<1	5	*	*	*	4
110	N.A.	0	2	*	*	4	2
430	430	4	11	2	8	15	30
280	60	1	3	*	*	8	25
720	65	1	4	2	4	6	2
80	30	0	1	*	*	*	*
240	25	0	2	*	*	2	15
300	10	<1	2	*	*	*	*
0	40	<1	2	N.A.	N.A.	N.A.	N.A.
10	70	<1	4	N.A.	N.A.	N.A.	N.A.
90	0	0	<1	N.A.	N.A.	N.A.	N.A.

∽ CONDIMENTS

	Calories	Saturated fat (g)	Polyunsaturated fat (g)	Total fat (g)	Calories from fat	Cholesterol (mg)
Newburg sauce with sherry, Snow's, canned, ⅓ cup	120	N.A.	N.A.	8	70	N.A.
Olives						
green pickled, 10 medium	50	<1	N.A.	5	45	0
black ripe, 10 medium	70	<1	N.A.	8	70	0
black ripe, salt-cured (Greek), 10 medium	90	1	N.A.	9	80	0
Onions, sweet, Heinz, jarred, 1 onion	40	0	0	0	0	N.A.
Pasta sauce (*see* Spaghetti sauce, below)						
Peppers, canned or jarred						
Heinz, 1 pepper or slice, hot and sweet	6	0	0	0	0	N.A.
Progresso, roasted, ½ cup	20	<1	<1	<1	N.A.	0
sweet fried, ½ jar	40	<1	<1	3	25	0
Picante sauce						
Old El Paso, 2 tbsp	8	N.A.	N.A.	<1	N.A.	0
Wise, 2 tbsp	12	0	0	0	0	N.A.
Pickles, dill, Heinz, 1 oz, all varieties	4	0	0	0	0	N.A.
sweet, 1 oz, all varieties	30	0	0	0	0	N.A.
Pizza sauce, Ragu, 3 tbsp	25	N.A.	N.A.	1	10	0
Pizza Quick, 3 tbsp	35	N.A.	N.A.	2	18	0
Plum sauce, tangy, La Choy, 1 tbsp	25	N.A.	N.A.	<1	N.A.	0
Relishes, Heinz, 1 oz, all varieties	35	0	0	0	0	N.A.
Salsas, Old El Paso						
green chili salsa, 2 tbsp	4	0	0	0	0	0
medium, hot, 2 tbsp	6	N.A.	N.A.	<1	N.A.	0
picante salsa, 2 tbsp	10	N.A.	N.A.	<1	N.A.	N.A.
salsa verde, 2 tbsp	10	0	0	<1	N.A.	0
thick 'n chunky, 2 tbsp	6	N.A.	N.A.	<1	N.A.	0
Salt, 1 tsp	0	0	0	0	0	N.A.

*Less than 2% U.S. RDA

Sodium (mg)	Potassium (mg)	Protein (g)	Carbohydrate (g)	Calcium (% U.S. RDA)	Iron (% U.S. RDA)	Vitamin A (% U.S. RDA)	Vitamin C (% U.S. RDA)
520	110	3	10	8	2	2	*
940	20	0	1	2	6	2	N.A.
290	10	0	1	4	6	*	N.A.
850	N.A.	1	2	N.A.	N.A.	N.A.	N.A.
170	N.A.	0	9	*	*	N.A.	N.A.
310	N.A.	0	1	2	*	N.A.	N.A.
0	160	<1	5	*	6	45	340
15	110	<1	4	*	4	8	160
310	70	<1	2	*	*	2	*
130	65	0	3	*	*	15	*
320	N.A.	0	<1	*	*	N.A.	N.A.
200	N.A.	0	7	*	*	N.A.	N.A.
200	N.A.	1	3	*	*	6	8
330	N.A.	1	3	*	2	6	6
10	10	<1	6	*	*	*	*
220	N.A.	0	8	*	*	N.A.	N.A.
270	15	0	1	*	*	*	*
170	N.A.	<1	<1	*	*	4	2
160	N.A.	<1	2	*	*	10	2
135	90	<1	2	*	*	2	10
170	N.A.	<1	1	*	*	4	2
2300	0	0	0	N.A.	N.A.	N.A.	N.A.

~ CONDIMENTS

	Calories	Saturated fat (g)	Polyunsat-urated fat (g)	Total fat (g)	Calories from fat	Choles-terol (mg)
Soy sauce, 1 tbsp (La Choy lite soy sauce contains 660 mg sodium)	10	0	0	0	0	0
Spaghetti sauce						
alfredo, Progresso Authentic, ½ cup	340	19	1	30	270	95
clam, Progresso, white, ½ cup	110	N.A.	N.A.	8	70	N.A.
red, ½ cup	70	N.A.	N.A.	3	25	N.A.
Classico (International Gourmet), ½ cup, D'Abruzzi	110	N.A.	N.A.	11	100	10
Di Bologna, Di Napoli, Di Roma Arrabbiata, Di Sicilia, DiVeneto	60	N.A.	N.A.	3	25	6
marinara, Progresso Authentic, ½ cup	110	2	<1	6	50	4
meat, Hunt's, ½ cup	70	<1	<1	2	18	2
meat-flavored, Prego, ½ cup	150	N.A.	N.A.	6	50	N.A.
mushroom varieties, Prego Extra Chunky, ½ cup (no-salt-added varieties contain 25 mg sodium)	110	N.A.	N.A.	6	50	N.A.
seafood, Progresso Authentic, ½ cup	190	9	<1	15	140	95
Sicilian, Progresso Authentic, ½ cup	30	<1	<1	3	25	0
Sweet and sour sauce, La Choy, 1 tbsp	25	N.A.	N.A.	<1	N.A.	0
Szechwan sauce, La Choy, hot and spicy, 1 tbsp	25	N.A.	N.A.	<1	N.A.	0
Taco dip						
Old El Paso, 2 tbsp	14	N.A.	N.A.	<1	N.A.	N.A.
Wise, 2 tbsp	12	0	0	0	0	N.A.
Taco sauce, Old El Paso, 2 tbsp canned	16	0	0	0	0	0
2 tbsp from jar (mild, medium, hot)	10	N.A.	N.A.	<1	N.A.	0

*Less than 2% U.S. RDA

Sodium (mg)	Potassium (mg)	Protein (g)	Carbohy-drate (g)	Calcium (% U.S. RDA)	Iron (% U.S. RDA)	Vitamin A (% U.S. RDA)	Vitamin C (% U.S. RDA)
1030	65	2	2	*	4	*	*
1080	70	13	6	40	2	30	*
280	65	9	1	*	2	*	4
560	210	5	7	2	4	8	*
600	N.A.	3	<1	2	2	4	4
340	N.A.	1	6	4	4	10	15
250	470	4	10	8	10	20	30
570	650	2	12	*	10	15	30
670	N.A.	2	20	2	6	20	25
490	N.A.	1	13	*	6	10	20
570	125	7	5	4	4	15	*
660	80	<1	2	2	2	*	2
190	5	<1	7	*	*	*	*
70	5	<1	6	*	*	*	4
75	75	0	3	*	*	*	*
115	85	0	3	*	*	15	*
300	150	1	3	*	2	4	10
130	N.A.	<1	2	*	*	*	2

∾ CONDIMENTS

	Calories	Saturated fat (g)	Polyunsaturated fat (g)	Total fat (g)	Calories from fat	Cholesterol (mg)
Teriyaki sauce, 1 tbsp	16	0	0	0	0	0
Tomato sauce, canned, 1 cup (no-salt-added varieties contain 40 mg sodium)	70	<1	<1	<1	N.A.	0
with herbs & cheese, 1 cup	140	<1	2	5	45	N.A.
with mushrooms, 1 cup	90	<1	<1	<1	N.A.	0
Spanish style, 1 cup	80	<1	<1	<1	N.A.	0
Vinegar, cider, 1 tbsp	2	0	0	0	0	N.A.
Worcestershire sauce, Heinz, 1 tbsp	10	N.A.	N.A.	N.A.	N.A.	N.A.
Yeast, active dry, Fleishmann's						
compressed, 1 cube	15	0	0	0	0	N.A.
nutritional, 1 oz	80	N.A.	N.A.	<1	N.A.	N.A.
regular or rapid rise, 1 packet	20	0	0	0	0	N.A.

*Less than 2% U.S. RDA

Sodium (mg)	Potassium (mg)	Protein (g)	Carbohy-drate (g)	Calcium (% U.S. RDA)	Iron (% U.S. RDA)	Vitamin A (% U.S. RDA)	Vitamin C (% U.S. RDA)
690	40	1	3	*	2	*	*
1480	910	3	18	4	15	50	50
N.A.	N.A.	5	25	10	15	50	40
1110	930	4	21	4	15	45	50
1150	N.A.	4	18	4	60	50	35
0	15	0	<1	*	*	N.A.	N.A.
230	N.A.	N.A.	N.A.	N.A.	N.A.	N.A.	N.A.
5	100	2	2	N.A.	N.A.	N.A.	N.A.
0	580	11	11	10	35	*	*
10	150	3	3	N.A.	N.A.	N.A.	N.A.

CRACKERS

CHIPS

& OTHER SNACKS

These are listed alphabetically by product name or type. Fiber values are scarce but have been included where available. Sugar values are not readily available yet for these products.

～ CRACKERS, CHIPS & OTHER SNACKS	Calories	Saturated fat (g)	Polyunsat-urated fat (g)	Total fat (g)	Calories from fat	Choles-terol (mg)
American Classic Crackers (Nabisco), ½ oz (4 crackers), all varieties	70	<1	<1	4	35	1
American Heritage (Sunshine), ½ oz (4 crackers) (sesame, wheat bran)	70	1	<1	4	35	0
Bacon Flavored Thins (Nabisco), ½ oz (7 crackers)	70	1	<1	4	35	1
Better Cheddars (Nabisco), ½ oz (10 crackers) (low-salt contains 65 mg sodium)	70	<1	<1	4	35	1
Bran Thins (Nabisco), ½ oz (7 crackers)	60	<1	<1	3	25	0
Bravos (Wise), 1 oz	150	N.A.	N.A.	8	70	N.A.
Bugles (General Mills), 1 oz (⅙ pkg) (regular, nacho cheese)	160	N.A.	N.A.	9	80	N.A.
Butter Flavored Thin Crackers (Pepperidge Farm), 4 crackers	70	1	0	3	25	3
Cereal bars (see Breakfast Cereals)						
Cheddar Wedges (Nabisco), ½ oz (31 crackers)	70	<1	<1	3	25	1
Cheese Sandwich Crackers, 1 oz (4 sandwiches) (regular, peanut butter)	140	1	2	7	60	0
Cheese Nips (Nabisco), ½ oz (13 crackers)	70	<1	<1	3	25	1
Cheese Shuffles (Sunshine), ½ oz (18 crackers)	70	1	<1	3	25	1
Cheez Balls (Planters), 1 oz	160	2	1	10	90	5
Cheez Doodles, puffed (Wise), 1 oz baked	150	N.A.	N.A.	9	80	N.A.
crunchy, 1 oz fried	160	N.A.	N.A.	10	90	N.A.
Cheez Waffles (Wise), 1 oz	140	N.A.	N.A.	8	70	N.A.

*Less than 2% U.S. RDA

Sodium (mg)	Potassium (mg)	Protein (g)	Carbohy-drate (g)	Dietary fiber (g)	Calcium (% U.S. RDA)	Iron (% U.S. RDA)	Vitamin A (% U.S. RDA)	Vitamin C (% U.S. RDA)
130	N.A.	1	9	N.A.	*	4	*	*
130	N.A.	2	8	N.A.	*	2	*	*
210	N.A.	1	9	N.A.	*	2	*	*
130	N.A.	2	8	N.A.	*	2	*	*
70	N.A.	1	9	N.A.	*	4	*	*
180	55	2	18	N.A.	4	2	*	*
270	30	2	18	N.A.	*	6	*	*
115	N.A.	1	10	N.A.	*	*	*	*
240	N.A.	1	9	N.A.	*	4	*	*
300	85	4	17	N.A.	2	4	*	*
130	N.A.	1	9	N.A.	2	2	*	*
140	N.A.	2	8	N.A.	2	2	*	*
290	45	2	15	N.A.	*	*	*	*
360	70	2	16	N.A.	2	*	*	*
230	50	2	16	N.A.	2	*	*	*
420	180	3	14	N.A.	6	2	*	*

~ CRACKERS, CHIPS & OTHER SNACKS	Calories	Saturated fat (g)	Polyunsaturated fat (g)	Total fat (g)	Calories from fat	Cholesterol (mg)
Cheez-it (Sunshine), ½ oz (12 crackers) (low-salt contains 65 mg sodium)	70	1	<1	4	35	1
Chex Snack Mix (Ralston), 1 oz (⅔ cup), all varieties (barbeque flavor contains 480 mg sodium)	120	N.A.	N.A.	5	45	0
Chicken in a Biskit (Nabisco), ½ oz (7 crackers)	80	1	<1	5	45	1
Club Crackers (Keebler), ½ oz (4 crackers) (low-salt contains 75 mg sodium)	60	<1	<1	3	25	0
Club & Cheddar Crackers (Keebler), ½ oz (1 cracker)	70	<1	<1	4	35	3
Clubettes (Keebler), ½ oz (22 combined crackers)	70	<1	<1	4	35	0
Combos (Mars), pretzel, 1.8 oz	240	N.A.	N.A.	9	80	N.A.
cracker Combos, 1 oz, all flavors	140	N.A.	N.A.	7	60	N.A.
Corn Cakes (Quaker), 1 cake	35	0	0	0	0	N.A.
Corn chips						
Frito-Lay Fritos, 1 oz (34 chips)	150	N.A.	N.A.	9	80	0
Health Valley, 1 oz unsalted	160	N.A.	N.A.	11	100	0
Corn Crisps (Pringle's), 1 oz (fresh roasted, tangy cheese)	140	N.A.	N.A.	7	60	0
Corn Snackers (Weight Watchers), 1 bag (½ oz), lightly salted (nacho cheese flavor contains 240 mg sodium)	60	N.A.	N.A.	2	18	N.A.
Corn Spirals/Twists (Wise), 1 oz (nacho cheese flavor contains 190 mg sodium)	160	N.A.	N.A.	10	90	N.A.
Cracker Jack (Borden), 1 oz (⅔ cup)	120	N.A.	N.A.	3	25	N.A.

*Less than 2% U.S. RDA

Sodium (mg)	Potassium (mg)	Protein (g)	Carbohy-drate (g)	Dietary fiber (g)	Calcium (% U.S. RDA)	Iron (% U.S. RDA)	Vitamin A (% U.S. RDA)	Vitamin C (% U.S. RDA)
135	N.A.	2	7	N.A.	2	2	*	*
310	N.A.	3	19	N.A.	*	25	*	10
130	N.A.	1	8	N.A.	*	2	*	*
150	20	1	9	N.A.	*	2	*	*
115	50	1	7	N.A.	*	2	*	*
150	20	1	9	N.A.	*	2	*	*
580	N.A.	5	34	N.A.	8	6	*	*
250	115	3	16	N.A.	4	4	*	*
50	15	1	7	0.2	*	*	*	*
220	50	2	16	N.A.	2	*	*	*
0	30	1	15	1	*	2	2	*
210	N.A.	2	17	N.A.	*	2	6	2
190	N.A.	1	10	N.A.	2	2	*	*
125	40	2	15	N.A.	2	2	*	*
90	115	2	22	N.A.	2	2	*	*

CRACKERS, CHIPS & OTHER SNACKS	Calories	Saturated fat (g)	Polyunsat-urated fat (g)	Total fat (g)	Calories from fat	Choles-terol (mg)
Crown Pilot (Nabisco), ½ oz (1 cracker)	70	<1	<1	2	18	1
Doo Dads (Nabisco), 1 oz (¹⁄₁₀ of pkg)	140	N.A.	N.A.	6	50	N.A.
English Water Biscuit (Pepper-idge Farm), 4 crackers	70	0	0	1	10	0
Escort (Nabisco), ½ oz (3 crackers)	70	<1	<1	4	35	0
Fiber Crisp (Fantastic Foods), 1 slice	50	N.A.	N.A.	<1	N.A.	N.A.
Formulated nuts (wheat based), 1 oz	180	3	7	18	160	0
Graham crackers and crumbs (see Desserts)						
Great Snackers (Weight Watchers), 1 pouch (½ oz), all varieties	60	N.A.	N.A.	3	25	N.A.
Harvest Crisps (Nabisco), ½ oz (6 crackers) (oat, 5-grain)	60	<1	<1	2	18	0
Harvest Wheats (Keebler), ½ oz (4 crackers)	60	<1	<1	3	25	0
Hi Ho Crackers (Sunshine), ½ oz (4 crackers) (low-salt contains 60 mg sodium)	80	1	1	5	45	0
whole wheat, ½ oz	70	1	<1	3	25	0
Meal Mates (Nabisco), ½ oz (3 wafers)	70	<1	<1	3	25	0
Nuts (see Legumes & Seeds)						
Oat Bran Crackers (Sunshine), ½ oz (8 crackers)	80	1	<1	4	35	0
Oat Bran Krisp Crackers (Ral-ston), ½ oz (2 triple crack-ers)	60	N.A.	N.A.	3	25	0
Oat Thins (Nabisco), ½ oz (8 crackers)	70	<1	<1	3	25	0

*Less than 2% U.S. RDA

Sodium (mg)	Potassium (mg)	Protein (g)	Carbohy-drate (g)	Dietary fiber (g)	Calcium (% U.S. RDA)	Iron (% U.S. RDA)	Vitamin A (% U.S. RDA)	Vitamin C (% U.S. RDA)
70	N.A.	1	11	N.A.	*	4	*	*
360	N.A.	3	18	N.A.	2	4	*	*
100	N.A.	2	13	N.A.	*	2	*	*
115	N.A.	1	9	N.A.	*	2	*	*
110	N.A.	2	11	4.9	N.A.	N.A.	N.A.	N.A.
25	90	4	6	N.A.	*	4	N.A.	N.A.
150	N.A.	1	8	N.A.	*	2	*	*
135	N.A.	1	10	N.A.	2	4	*	*
95	25	1	8	N.A.	*	2	*	*
130	N.A.	1	8	N.A.	*	2	*	*
130	N.A.	1	8	N.A.	*	2	*	*
160	N.A.	1	9	N.A.	2	2	*	*
140	N.A.	1	9	N.A.	*	2	*	*
140	N.A.	1	9	3	N.A.	2	N.A.	N.A.
90	N.A.	1	10	N.A.	*	2	*	*

~ CRACKERS, CHIPS & OTHER SNACKS	Calories	Saturated fat (g)	Polyunsat-urated fat (g)	Total fat (g)	Calories from fat	Choles-terol (mg)
Onion Flavored Rings (Wise), 1 oz	130	N.A.	N.A.	5	45	N.A.
Oyster crackers (see Soup crackers, below)						
Pizza Rolls, Jeno's (Pillsbury), 3 oz (6 rolls), cheese	240	N.A.	N.A.	12	110	N.A.
Popcorn, 3 cups popped, plain	70	N.A.	N.A.	<1	N.A.	N.A.
General Mills Pop-Secret, 3 cups popped (¼ pkg), (natural, butter)	100	2	<1	6	50	0
cheese flavor, 2¾ cups as packaged (⅓ pkg)	170	N.A.	N.A.	11	100	0
light, 3 cups popped	70	<1	<1	3	25	0
salt-free butter flavor, 3 cups as packaged (⅓ pkg)	140	N.A.	N.A.	9	80	0
Orville Redenbacher's Gourmet, 3 cups original, white (hot-air variety contains 40 calories and <1 gram fat)	80	N.A.	N.A.	4	35	0
Popping and Topping, 1 tbsp	120	2	8	14	130	0
Popcorn, Microwave						
Orville Redenbacher's Gourmet, 3 cups popped (regular and frozen, natural and butter flavor) (salt-free contains 0 mg sodium)	80	1	<1	5	45	0
butter toffee, caramel	230	3	1	13	120	<1
cheddar cheese, nacho, sour cream 'n onion	130	2	<1	8	70	1
light	50	<1	<1	1	10	0
Pillsbury, 3 cups popped, frozen or shelf-stable (original & butter flavors)	210	N.A.	N.A.	13	120	N.A.
salt free	170	N.A.	N.A.	7	60	N.A.

*Less than 2% U.S. RDA

Sodium (mg)	Potassium (mg)	Protein (g)	Carbohy-drate (g)	Dietary fiber (g)	Calcium (% U.S. RDA)	Iron (% U.S. RDA)	Vitamin A (% U.S. RDA)	Vitamin C (% U.S. RDA)
360	45	<1	21	N.A.	2	2	*	*
350	95	8	23	N.A.	15	10	6	2
0	N.A.	2	14	N.A.	*	*	N.A.	N.A.
170	60	2	11	2	*	2	*	*
260	60	3	15	2	2	2	*	*
140	N.A.	2	12	2	*	2	*	*
0	60	2	16	2	*	2	*	*
0	60	1	10	3	*	2	*	*
0	0	0	0	0	N.A.	N.A.	N.A.	N.A.
210	60	2	9	3	*	2	*	*
90	125	2	28	2	*	6	6	*
310	85	2	14	2.7	*	*	*	*
80	60	2	9	3	*	2	*	*
440	95	3	20	N.A.	*	2	*	4
0	110	3	23	N.A.	*	4	*	4

~ CRACKERS, CHIPS & OTHER SNACKS	Calories	Saturated fat (g)	Polyunsaturated fat (g)	Total fat (g)	Calories from fat	Cholesterol (mg)
Popcorn Cake (Riceland), 1 cake	35	N.A.	N.A.	<1	N.A.	0
Potato chips, 1 oz (14 chips)	150	3	5	10	90	0
made from dry potatoes, 1 oz	160	4	<1	13	120	0
Light (Frito-Lay), 0.9 oz (18 chips)	120	N.A.	N.A.	6	50	0
Pretzels, Bachman, 1 oz (nutzels, logs, buttertwist, petite) (hard pretzels contain <1 g fat and 290 mg sodium)	110	N.A.	N.A.	2	18	0
Rice cake, 1 cake, all varieties (salt-free varieties contain 0 mg sodium)	40	N.A.	N.A.	<1	N.A.	0
Ritz (Nabisco) ½ oz (4 crackers) (low-salt contains 60 mg sodium)	70	<1	<1	4	35	1
Ritz Bits (Nabisco), ½ oz (22 crackers) (low-salt contains 60 mg sodium; cheese contains <2 mg cholesterol and 150 mg sodium)	70	<1	<1	4	35	0
Ritz Bits Sandwiches (Nabisco), ½ oz (6 sandwiches), cheese	80	1	<1	5	45	1
peanut butter	80	<1	<1	4	35	0
Royal Lunch (Nabisco), ½ oz (1 cracker)	60	<1	<1	2	18	3
Rye Cakes (Quaker), 1 cake	35	0	0	0	0	0
Ry-Krisp (Ralston), ½ oz (2 triple crackers), all varieties	45	N.A.	N.A.	1	10	0
Saltine crackers, ½ oz (5 crackers) (low-salt contains 105 mg sodium; unsalted tops contain 115 mg sodium)	60	<1	<1	2	18	0
fat-free (Nabisco)	50	0	0	0	0	0
whole wheat (Sunshine)	60	<1	<1	1	10	0

*Less than 2% U.S. RDA

Sodium (mg)	Potassium (mg)	Protein (g)	Carbohy-drate (g)	Dietary fiber (g)	Calcium (% U.S. RDA)	Iron (% U.S. RDA)	Vitamin A (% U.S. RDA)	Vitamin C (% U.S. RDA)
25	20	1	7	N.A.	*	*	*	*
135	370	2	15 .	N.A.	*	*	*	10
220	310	2	12	N.A.	*	2	N.A.	4
170	410	1	17	N.A.	*	*	*	8
440	40	3	21	N.A.	*	10	*	*
30	25	1	7	0.3	*	*	*	*
120	N.A.	1	9	N.A.	2	2	*	*
120	N.A.	1	9	N.A.	2	2	*	*
135	N.A.	1	7	N.A.	2	2	*	*
80	N.A.	2	8	N.A.	2	2	*	*
80	N.A.	1	10	N.A.	2	2	*	*
50	45	1	7	0.8	*	4	*	*
105	65	1	11	3.2	*	2	*	*
190	20	1	10	N.A.	*	2	*	*
115	N.A.	1	12	N.A.	*	4	*	*
210 .	N.A.	1	10	1	*	4	*	*

∿ CRACKERS, CHIPS & OTHER SNACKS	Calories	Saturated fat (g)	Polyunsaturated fat (g)	Total fat (g)	Calories from fat	Cholesterol (mg)
Sesame Crackers (Pepperidge Farm), 4 crackers	80	1	0	4	35	0
Snack Sticks (Pepperidge Farm), 8 crackers, all varieties	140	1	1	5	45	0
Sociables (Nabisco), ½ oz (6 crackers)	70	<1	<1	3	25	1
Soup crackers, ½ oz, about 18 crackers	60	<1	<1	2	18	0
Swiss Cheese Crackers (Nabisco), ½ oz (7 crackers)	70	<1	<1	3	25	1
Tato Skins (Keebler), 1 oz, all flavors	150	1	1	8	70	0
Thin Bits (Keebler), ½ oz (12 crackers)	70	<1	<1	3	25	0
Tid Bits (Nabisco), ½ oz (16 crackers)	70	1	<1	4	35	1
Toast Crackers (Planters), 1 oz (4 sandwiches)	140	2	3	7	60	0
Toasteds (Keebler), ½ oz (4 crackers)	60	<1	<1	3	25	0
Tortilla chips, 1 oz (15–16 chips), all varieties (unsalted contains 5 mg sodium)	150	N.A.	N.A.	8	70	0
Town House Crackers (Keebler), ½ oz (9 crackers)	70	<1	<1	4	35	0
Triscuit (Nabisco), ½ oz (3 regular crackers, 8 Bits crackers) (low-salt contains 35 mg sodium)	60	<1	<1	2	18	0
Twigs (Nabisco), ½ oz (5 pieces)	70	<1	<1	4	35	1
Uneeda Biscuits (Nabisco), ½ oz (2 biscuits)	60	<1	<1	2	18	0
Vegetable Thins (Nabisco), ½ oz (7 crackers)	70	<1	<1	4	35	1

*Less than 2% U.S. RDA

Sodium (mg)	Potassium (mg)	Protein (g)	Carbohy-drate (g)	Dietary fiber (g)	Calcium (% U.S. RDA)	Iron (% U.S. RDA)	Vitamin A (% U.S. RDA)	Vitamin C (% U.S. RDA)
140	N.A.	2	12	2	*	2	*	*
340	N.A.	4	19	N.A.	4	4	*	*
135	N.A.	1	9	N.A.	2	2	*	*
180	20	1	10	N.A.	*	4	*	*
170	N.A.	1	11	N.A.	2	2	*	*
170	230	1	17	N.A.	*	2	*	*
50	15	1	10	N.A.	*	2	*	*
200	N.A.	1	8	N.A.	2	2	*	*
270	85	4	15	N.A.	2	4	*	*
135	20	1	9	N.A.	*	2	*	*
180	60	2	18	0.5	4	2	*	*
120	10	1	8	N.A.	*	2	*	*
75	N.A.	1	10	N.A.	*	2	*	*
140	N.A.	1	8	N.A.	4	2	*	*
100	N.A.	1	10	N.A.	*	4	*	*
140	N.A.	1	8	N.A.	2	2	*	*

~ CRACKERS, CHIPS & OTHER SNACKS	Calories	Saturated fat (g)	Polyunsat- urated fat (g)	Total fat (g)	Calories from fat	Choles- terol (mg)
Waverly Wafers (Nabisco), ½ oz (4 crackers) (low-salt contains 80 mg sodium)	70	<1	<1	3	25	0
Wheat Cakes (Quaker), 1 cake	35	0	0	0	0	0
Wheat Crackers (Pepperidge Farm), 4 crackers, hearty	100	1	0	5	45	0
Wheat Crackers, Stoned (Health Valley), 1 oz (regu- lar, sesame)	130	N.A.	N.A.	5	45	0
Wheats, Sun Toasted (Kee- bler), ½ oz (10 crackers)	70	<1	<1	4	35	0
Wheat Thins (Nabisco), ½ oz (8 crackers) (regular, nutty) (low-salt contains 60 mg sodium)	70	<1	<1	4	35	0
Wheats Snack Crackers (Sun- shine), ½ oz (8 crackers)	70	1	<1	4	35	0
Wheatables (Keebler), ½ oz (12 crackers) (regular, white cheddar) (low-salt contains 70 mg sodium)	70	<1	1	4	35	0
Wheatsworth (Nabisco), ½ oz (4 crackers)	70	<1	<1	3	25	0
Zweiback Toast (Nabisco), ½ oz (2 pieces)	60	<1	<1	1	10	1

*Less than 2% U.S. RDA

Sodium (mg)	Potassium (mg)	Protein (g)	Carbohy-drate (g)	Dietary fiber (g)	Calcium (% U.S. RDA)	Iron (% U.S. RDA)	Vitamin A (% U.S. RDA)	Vitamin C (% U.S. RDA)
160	N.A.	1	10	N.A.	*	2	*	*
50	45	1	7	0.8	*	2	*	*
140	N.A.	2	13	1	*	2	*	*
40	115	3	17	3.2	*	4	*	*
105	20	1	8	N.A.	2	4	*	*
160	N.A.	1	9	N.A.	*	2	*	*
170	N.A.	1	9	N.A.	*	2	*	*
140	50	1	9	N.A.	*	2	*	*
135	N.A.	1	9	N.A.	*	4	*	*
20	N.A.	2	10	N.A.	*	2	*	*

~ DAIRY PRODUCTS
~ & EGGS

~ *This includes cheeses as well as milk, yogurt, and ice cream. Egg and milk substitutes are also listed. The sugar lactose is present in milk products, but listings for it are not widely available. Dairy products are not a source of fiber.*

~ DAIRY PRODUCTS & EGGS	Calories	Saturated fat (g)	Polyunsaturated fat (g)	Total fat (g)	Calories from fat	Cholesterol (mg)
Breakfast Mix, Instant, Pillsbury, 1 pouch prepared, all flavors	300	N.A.	N.A.	9	80	N.A.
Butter						
regular, 1 tsp (unsalted contains 0 mg sodium)	35	3	<1	4	35	11
1 stick (8 tbsp) (unsalted stick contains 12 mg sodium)	810	57	3	92	830	248
whipped, 1 tsp	25	2	<1	3	25	8
1 stick (8 tbsp)	540	38	2	60	540	165
Cheese, natural						
blue, 1 oz	100	5	<1	8	70	21
brick, 1 oz	110	5	<1	8	70	27
brie, 1 oz	100	N.A.	N.A.	8	70	28
camembert, 1 oz	90	4	<1	7	60	20
chedarella, Land O Lakes, 1 oz	100	5	<1	8	70	25
cheddar, 1 oz	110	6	<1	9	80	30
light, Cabot Vitalait, 1 oz	70	N.A.	N.A.	5	45	15
reduced fat, Kraft, 1 oz	90	3	0	5	45	20
colby, 1 oz	110	6	<1	9	80	27
Weight Watchers, 1 oz	80	2	0	5	45	15
cream cheese, 1 oz	100	6	<1	10	90	31
slice, Kraft, 1.2 oz	120	N.A.	N.A.	12	110	N.A.
light, Kraft, 1 oz	60	N.A.	N.A.	5	45	10
edam, 1 oz	100	5	<1	8	70	25
feta, 1 oz	80	4	<1	6	50	25
gouda, 1 oz	100	5	<1	8	70	32
grated, Progresso, 1 tbsp (Romano, Parmesan)	25	1	<1	2	18	5
Gruyère, 1 oz	120	5	<1	9	80	31
limburger, 1 oz	90	5	<1	8	70	26
Monterey Jack, 1 oz	110	N.A.	N.A.	9	80	N.A.

*Less than 2% U.S. RDA

Sodium (mg)	Potassium (mg)	Protein (g)	Carbohy-drate (g)	Calcium (% U.S. RDA)	Iron (% U.S. RDA)	Vitamin A (% U.S. RDA)	Vitamin C (% U.S. RDA)
320	610	14	40	25	25	30	30
40	0	<1	0	*	*	4	*
940	30	1	<1	2	*	70	*
30	0	0	0	*	*	2	*
630	20	<1	N.A.	2	*	45	*
400	75	6	<1	15	*	4	*
160	40	7	<1	20	*	6	*
180	45	6	<1	6	*	4	*
240	55	6	<1	10	*	6	*
180	20	7	<1	20	*	6	*
180	30	7	<1	20	*	6	*
170	N.A.	8	1	25	*	4	*
200	N.A.	8	1	25	*	6	*
170	35	7	<1	20	*	6	*
130	N.A.	8	1	25	*	4	*
85	35	2	<1	2	2	8	*
170	N.A.	2	1	2	*	4	*
160	N.A.	3	2	4	*	6	*
270	55	7	<1	20	*	6	*
320	20	4	1	15	*	N.A.	*
230	35	7	<1	20	*	4	*
75	5	2	<1	6	*	*	*
95	25	9	<1	30	N.A.	6	*
230	35	6	<1	15	*	8	*
150	25	7	<1	20	*	6	*

DAIRY PRODUCTS & EGGS	Calories	Saturated fat (g)	Polyunsaturated fat (g)	Total fat (g)	Calories from fat	Cholesterol (mg)
Weight Watchers, 1 oz	80	2	0	5	45	15
mozzarella, 1 oz	80	4	<1	6	50	22
part skim, 1 oz	70	3	<1	5	45	16
low-moisture, 1 oz	90	4	<1	7	60	25
part skim, 1 oz	80	3	<1	5	45	15
Weight Watchers, 1 oz	70	2	0	4	35	15
muenster, 1 oz	100	5	<1	9	80	27
Neufchâtel, 1 oz	70	4	<1	7	60	22
hard, 1 oz	110	5	<1	7	60	19
Port du Salut, 1 oz	100	5	<1	8	70	35
provolone, 1 oz	100	5	<1	8	70	20
ricotta, ½ cup, whole milk	220	10	<1	16	140	63
part skim, ½ cup	170	6	<1	10	90	38
roquefort, 1 oz	110	6	<1	9	80	26
Swiss, 1 oz	110	5	<1	8	70	26
Weight Watchers, 1 oz	90	2	0	5	45	15
Cheese, process slices, 1-oz slice (American, cheddar, Swiss)	110	6	<1	8	70	27
Cheese product						
Borden Lite-Line, 1-oz slice (American, mozzarella, sharp cheddar, Swiss)	50	N.A.	N.A.	2	18	N.A.
Lite-Line Sodium Lite (reduced sodium variety contains 90 mg sodium)	70	N.A.	N.A.	4	35	N.A.
Kraft Light singles, 1 oz	70	3	0	4	35	15
Shedd's Country Crock, cold pack, 1 oz	70	N.A.	N.A.	4	35	15
Sargento, shredded, 1 oz	90	N.A.	N.A.	7	60	0
Velveeta Light (Kraft), block, 1 oz	70	2	0	4	35	15
Weight Watchers American, 1-oz slice (low-sodium contains 120 mg sodium)	50	1	0	2	18	5

*Less than 2% U.S. RDA

Sodium (mg)	Potassium (mg)	Protein (g)	Carbohy-drate (g)	Calcium (% U.S. RDA)	Iron (% U.S. RDA)	Vitamin A (% U.S. RDA)	Vitamin C (% U.S. RDA)
120	N.A.	8	1	25	*	4	*
105	20	6	<1	15	*	4	*
130	25	7	<1	20	*	4	*
120	20	6	<1	15	*	6	*
150	25	8	<1	20	*	4	*
120	N.A.	8	1	25	*	4	*
180	40	7	<1	20	*	6	*
115	30	3	<1	2	*	6	*
450	25	10	<1	35	*	4	*
150	N.A.	7	<1	20	N.A.	8	*
250	40	7	<1	20	*	4	*
105	130	14	4	25	4	10	*
160	160	14	6	35	4	10	*
510	25	6	<1	20	*	6	*
75	30	8	1	25	*	4	*
40	N.A.	10	1	30	*	4	*
390	45	6	<1	20	*	6	*
390	35	7	1	20	*	*	*
200	360	6	2	20	*	2	*
420	N.A.	6	2	20	*	6	*
190	N.A.	5	2	20	*	4	*
280	N.A.	5	<1	20	*	6	*
450	N.A.	5	3	15	*	6	*
400	N.A.	6	2	20	*	4	*

~ DAIRY PRODUCTS & EGGS	Calories	Saturated fat (g)	Polyunsat- urated fat (g)	Total fat (g)	Calories from fat	Choles- terol (mg)
mild, sharp cheddar, 1-oz slice (low-sodium mild contains 70 mg sodium)	80	3	0	5	45	15
Swiss, 1-oz slice	50	1	0	2	18	5
Cheese, soy-based, 1 oz	70	1	<1	5	45	0
Cheese food, cold pack, 1 oz, American	90	4	<1	7	60	18
processed American, Swiss	90	4	<1	7	60	21
Cheese sauce						
canned Welsh Rarebit, Snow's, ½ cup	170	N.A.	N.A.	11	100	N.A.
refrigerated, Merkt's, 1 oz (13.2 oz jar)	80	N.A.	N.A.	6	50	15
Cheese spread, process Amer- ican, 1 oz	80	4	<1	6	50	16
Kraft Velveeta (block), 1 oz	80	N.A.	N.A.	6	50	N.A.
Kraft Velveeta slices, 1 oz	90	N.A.	N.A.	6	50	N.A.
Chocolate or carob-flavored powder, prepared with milk, 1 cup	220	5	<1	9	80	33
Cottage cheese						
creamed, 1 cup	220	6	<1	10	90	31
with fruit, 1 cup	280	5	<1	8	70	25
dry curd, unsalted, 1 cup	120	<1	0	<1	N.A.	10
2% lowfat, 1 cup	200	3	<1	4	35	19
1% lowfat, 1 cup	160	2	<1	2	18	10
Cream						
half & half, 1 tbsp	20	1	<1	2	18	6
heavy whipping cream, 1 cup (2 cups whipped)	820	55	3	88	790	326
light table cream, 1 tbsp	30	2	<1	3	25	10
light whipping cream, 1 cup (2 cups whipped)	700	46	2	74	670	270
sour						
cultured, 1 tbsp	25	2	<1	3	25	5

*Less than 2% U.S. RDA

Sodium (mg)	Potassium (mg)	Protein (g)	Carbohy-drate (g)	Calcium (% U.S. RDA)	Iron (% U.S. RDA)	Vitamin A (% U.S. RDA)	Vitamin C (% U.S. RDA)
150	N.A.	8	1	25	*	6	*
370	N.A.	7	2	20	*	*	*
140	N.A.	7	<1	20	*	6	*
270	105	6	2	15	*	4	*
390	80	6	2	20	*	6	*
460	25	9	10	25	2	10	*
260	N.A.	4	3	10	*	2	*
380	70	5	3	15	*	4	*
430	N.A.	5	2	15	*	4	*
390	N.A.	5	3	15	*	4	*
150	440	8	27	30	6	6	4
850	180	26	6	15	2	6	*
920	150	22	30	10	2	6	*
20	45	25	3	4	2	*	*
920	220	31	8	15	2	4	*
920	190	28	6	15	2	2	*
5	20	<1	<1	2	*	*	*
90	180	5	7	15	*	70	2
5	20	<1	<1	*	*	2	*
80	230	5	7	15	*	50	2
5	15	<1	<1	*	*	2	*

DAIRY PRODUCTS & EGGS	Calories	Saturated fat (g)	Polyunsaturated fat (g)	Total fat (g)	Calories from fat	Cholesterol (mg)
imitation, 1 oz	60	5	<1	6	50	0
light (Land O Lakes), 1 tbsp (with chives contains 150 mg sodium)	20	<1	<1	1	10	3
non-butterfat sour dressing, 1 tbsp	20	2	<1	2	18	1
Creamer						
dairy, instant nonfat dry milk, Weight Watchers, 1 packet	10	0	0	0	0	N.A.
non-dairy liquid frozen, ½ oz (1 tbsp)	20	<1	<1	2	18	0
powdered, 1 tsp	12	<1	<1	<1	N.A.	0
Dairy Light, Alba, 2.8 g	10	0	0	0	0	N.A.
Egg, raw, 1 large	80	2	<1	6	50	274
white only, 1 large	16	0	0	0	0	0
yolk only, 1 large	60	2	<1	6	50	272
Egg substitute						
Ener-G Egg Replacer, non-egg, 1½ tsp (1 egg)	16	0	0	0	0	0
Fleishmann's Egg Beaters, ¼ cup (1 egg)	25	0	0	0	0	0
Healthy Choice, ¼ cup	30	N.A.	N.A.	<1	N.A.	0
Scramblers (Morningstar Farms), ¼ cup	60	0	2	3	25	0
Tofutti Egg Watchers, ¼ cup	50	N.A.	N.A.	2	18	0
Eggnog						
canned, Borden, ¼ cup	160	N.A.	N.A.	9	80	N.A.
dairy, 1 cup	340	11	<1	19	170	149
powdered flavored mix, 2 tbsp	110	0	0	<1	N.A.	N.A.
Hot Chocolate Mix, Swiss Miss, ¾ cup prepared, all varieties	110	2	<1	3	25	2
Diet, ¾ cup	20	N.A.	N.A.	<1	N.A.	2

*Less than 2% U.S. RDA

Sodium (mg)	Potassium (mg)	Protein (g)	Carbohydrate (g)	Calcium (% U.S. RDA)	Iron (% U.S. RDA)	Vitamin A (% U.S. RDA)	Vitamin C (% U.S. RDA)
30	45	<1	2	*	N.A.	*	*
20	40	1	2	2	*	2	*
5	20	<1	<1	*	*	*	*
15	N.A.	1	1	4	*	*	*
10	30	<1	2	*	*	*	*
0	15	<1	1	*	*	*	*
15	N.A.	1	1	4	*	N.A.	N.A.
70	65	6	<1	2	6	6	*
50	45	3	<1	*	*	*	*
10	15	3	<1	2	6	6	*
0	0	0	3	4	*	*	*
80	N.A.	5	1	2	6	6	*
90	N.A.	5	1	*	4	10	*
130	70	6	3	4	4	20	*
100	N.A.	7	2	2	6	10	*
80	85	3	16	10	2	6	*
140	420	10	34	35	4	20	6
45	N.A.	<1	28	N.A.	2	N.A.	*
180	115	2	23	4	2	*	*
180	170	2	3	8	2	*	*

~ DAIRY PRODUCTS & EGGS	Calories	Saturated fat (g)	Polyunsat-urated fat (g)	Total fat (g)	Calories from fat	Choles-terol (mg)
Lite, ¾ cup	70	N.A.	N.A.	<1	N.A.	1
Sugar Free, ¾ cup	50	N.A.	N.A.	<1	N.A.	2
Ice cream						
light, 7% fat (Baskin-Robbins), ½ cup (4 oz), all flavors	120	3	2	5	45	10
no-fat (Sealtest Free), ½ cup	100	0	0	0	0	0
rich, 16% fat, 1 cup	350	15	<1	24	220	88
regular, 10% fat, 1 cup vanilla	270	9	<1	14	130	59
soft serve, 1 cup	380	14	1	23	210	153
sugar-free, 7% fat (Baskin-Robbins Low, Lite 'n Luscious), ½ cup (4 oz)	90	N.A.	N.A.	2	18	4
Ice cream bars and novelties						
Bakers Fudgetastic ice cream bar, all varieties	230	N.A.	N.A.	15	140	20
Eskimo Pie, 1 bar (3 oz)	180	N.A.	N.A.	12	110	N.A.
sugar free (2.5 oz)	140	N.A.	N.A.	12	110	N.A.
Haagen-Dazs ice cream bar, all varieties	340	N.A.	N.A.	24	220	N.A.
Jell-O pudding pops, all varieties	80	N.A.	N.A.	2	18	0
Kool-aid Kool Pops	40	0	0	0	0	0
Cream Pops	50	N.A.	N.A.	2	18	5
Weight Watchers chocolate dip bar	110	3	1	7	60	5
fudge bar, all varieties	60	N.A.	N.A.	<1	N.A.	5
vanilla sandwich bar	150	2	N.A.	3	25	5
Ice milk, hard, 1 cup	180	4	<1	6	50	18
soft serve, 1 cup	220	3	<1	5	45	13
Weight Watchers, ½ cup	110	2	0	4	35	8
Malted milk powder, 3 tsp (¾ oz), regular	90	<1	<1	2	18	4

*Less than 2% U.S. RDA

Sodium (mg)	Potassium (mg)	Protein (g)	Carbohy-drate (g)	Calcium (% U.S. RDA)	Iron (% U.S. RDA)	Vitamin A (% U.S. RDA)	Vitamin C (% U.S. RDA)
180	200	2	17	6	2	*	*
190	170	4	9	10	2	*	*
N.A.	N.A.	3	18	10	N.A.	N.A.	N.A.
45	N.A.	2	24	10	*	4	*
110	220	4	32	15	*	20	*
115	260	5	32	18	*	10	*
150	340	7	38	25	2	15	*
85	N.A.	3	18	10	N.A.	N.A.	N.A.
45	170	3	24	8	2	4	*
35	N.A.	2	16	6	2	4	*
35	N.A.	3	11	8	*	2	*
55	N.A.	4	30	N.A.	N.A.	N.A.	N.A.
80	75	2	13	8	*	*	*
10	0	0	10	*	*	*	10
20	30	1	9	2	*	*	10
35	N.A.	2	10	4	2	*	*
85	N.A.	3	12	8	*	*	*
170	N.A.	3	28	15	4	4	*
105	270	5	29	20	*	4	*
160	410	8	38	25	2	4	2
80	N.A.	4	18	10	*	*	*
95	160	3	15	6	*	*	*

～ DAIRY PRODUCTS & EGGS	Calories	Saturated fat (g)	Polyunsaturated fat (g)	Total fat (g)	Calories from fat	Cholesterol (mg)
chocolate	80	<1	<1	1	10	1
Margarines (see Fats, Oils, Margarines & Salad Dressings)						
Milk						
whole (3.7% fat), 1 cup	160	6	<1	9	80	35
low-sodium	150	5	<1	8	70	33
chocolate	210	5	<1	9	80	30
2% lowfat, 1 cup	120	3	<1	5	45	18
chocolate	180	3	<1	5	45	17
1% lowfat, 1 cup	100	2	<1	3	25	10
chocolate	160	2	<1	3	25	7
skim, 1 cup	90	<1	<1	<1	N.A.	4
buttermilk, cultured, 1 cup	100	1	<1	2	18	9
condensed sweetened (canned), 1 cup	980	17	1	27	240	104
dry nonfat, 1 cup	440	<1	<1	<1	N.A.	24
instant dry, 1 cup	240	<1	<1	<1	N.A.	12
reconstituted, Alba, 8 fluid oz	80	0	0	0	0	N.A.
evaporated whole (canned), ½ cup	170	6	<1	10	90	37
skim (canned), ½ cup	100	<1	<1	<1	N.A.	5
filled (canned), Pet, ½ cup	150	1	3	8	70	5
soy, ½ cup	40	<1	1	2	18	0
Milk shake, thick (11 oz)	360	6	<1	9	80	35
Milk shake mix, Alba Fit 'n Frosty, 1 envelope, all varieties	70	N.A.	N.A.	1	10	N.A.
MooTown Snackers (Sargento), 1 stick (8/10 oz)	70	N.A.	N.A.	4	35	15
Puddings (see Desserts)						
Sherbet, orange, 1 cup	270	2	<1	4	35	14

*Less than 2% U.S. RDA

Sodium (mg)	Potassium (mg)	Protein (g)	Carbohy-drate (g)	Calcium (% U.S. RDA)	Iron (% U.S. RDA)	Vitamin A (% U.S. RDA)	Vitamin C (% U.S. RDA)
50	130	1	18	*	2	*	N.A.
120	370	8	11	30	*	6	6
5	620	8	11	25	N.A.	6	N.A.
150	420	8	26	30	4	6	4
120	380	8	12	2	*	10	4
150	420	8	26	30	4	10	4
125	380	8	12	30	*	10	4
150	430	8	26	30	4	10	4
125	410	8	12	30	*	10	4
260	370	8	12	30	*	2	4
390	1140	24	167	90	4	20	15
640	2150	43	62	150	2	*	15
370	1160	24	36	80	*	30	6
190	N.A.	8	12	30	*	N.A.	N.A.
135	380	9	13	35	*	6	4
150	420	10	15	40	2	10	2
140	N.A.	8	12	30	*	10	4
15	170	3	2	*	4	*	*
320	620	11	60	45	4	8	*
200	N.A.	6	11	30	*	N.A.	N.A.
125	N.A.	7	<1	15	*	4	*
90	200	2	59	10	2	4	6

~ DAIRY PRODUCTS & EGGS	Calories	Saturated fat (g)	Polyunsat- urated fat (g)	Total fat (g)	Calories from fat	Choles- terol (mg)
Sorbet Fruit Whip, Baskin-Robbins, 4 oz	80	N.A.	N.A.	N.A.	N.A.	0
Sour cream (see Cream, sour, above)						
Tofutti, frozen soy dessert, ½ cup, all flavors	220	N.A.	N.A.	13	120	0
lite, 4 oz, all flavors	100	N.A.	N.A.	<1	N.A.	0
Topping, whipped						
frozen topping, 1 tbsp	14	<1	<1	1	10	0
1 cup	240	16	<1	19	170	0
powdered topping, non-dairy, 1 tbsp prepared	8	<1	<1	<1	N.A.	<1
1 cup	150	9	<1	10	90	8
Yogurt						
whole milk, 8 oz plain (1 cup)	140	5	<1	7	60	29
low-fat, 8 oz plain	140	2	<1	4	35	14
fruited low-fat, 8 oz	230	2	<1	3	25	10
nonfat, 8 oz plain	130	<1	<1	<1	N.A.	4
Weight Watchers Ultimate 90, 1 cup (8 oz)	90	N.A.	N.A.	<1	N.A.	5
Yoplait light, 6 oz	90	0	0	0	0	3
Yogurt, frozen						
low-fat, Baskin-Robbins, ½ cup	130	N.A.	N.A.	4	35	4
nonfat, Sealtest, ½ cup	100	0	0	0	0	0

*Less than 2% U.S. RDA

Sodium (mg)	Potassium (mg)	Protein (g)	Carbohy-drate (g)	Calcium (% U.S. RDA)	Iron (% U.S. RDA)	Vitamin A (% U.S. RDA)	Vitamin C (% U.S. RDA)
20	N.A.	0	24	*	N.A.	N.A.	N.A.
105	N.A.	3	22	*	2	*	*
120	N.A.	2	21	N.A.	N.A.	N.A.	N.A.
0	0	<1	<1	*	*	*	*
20	15	1	17	*	*	15	*
0	5	<1	<1	*	*	*	*
55	120	3	13	8	*	6	*
105	350	8	11	25	*	6	2
160	530	12	16	40	*	4	4
120	400	9	42	30	*	2	2
170	580	13	17	45	*	*	4
130	N.A.	10	13	35	*	*	*
100	370	7	14	25	*	*	*
40	N.A.	4	24	16	N.A.	N.A.	N.A.
35	N.A.	2	23	6	*	*	*

↜ DESSERTS

↝ *These are divided into cakes (including cupcakes, coffee cakes, doughnuts, and sweet rolls), cookies, gelatin, muffins, pies and pastries, and puddings. Products are listed by type and by product name. Listings for fiber and sugar content are not abundant enough to include.*

～ CAKES†

	Calories	Saturated fat (g)	Polyunsaturated fat (g)	Total fat (g)	Calories from fat	Cholesterol (mg)
Angel food cake mix, Betty Crocker, 1/12 cake	130	0	0	0	0	0
flavored varieties, 1/12 cake	150	0	0	0	0	0
Apple cinnamon cake mix, Betty Crocker, 1/12 cake	250	2	4	10	90	55
no cholesterol recipe, 1/12 cake	210	2	2	6	50	0
Apple 'n Spice Bake, Pepperidge Farm Dessert Light, 1 pkg	170	0	0	2	18	10
Apple streusel, Betty Crocker microwave cake mix, 1/6 cake	240	3	3	11	100	45
no cholesterol recipe, 1/6 cake	210	2	<1	8	70	0
Banana cake						
Pillsbury mix, 1/12 cake	250	N.A.	N.A.	11	100	N.A.
Sara Lee, iced single layer, 1/8 cake	170	N.A.	N.A.	6	50	N.A.
Black forest cake						
Pillsbury bundt mix, 1/16 cake	240	N.A.	N.A.	8	70	N.A.
Sara Lee two-layer, 1/8 cake	190	N.A.	N.A.	8	70	N.A.
Weight Watchers, 1/2 pkg	180	1	2	5	45	5
Boston cream pie						
Betty Crocker dessert mix, 1/8 pie	270	N.A.	N.A.	6	50	N.A.
Pepperidge Farm American Collection, 1 pkg	230	N.A.	N.A.	10	90	N.A.
Pillsbury bundt mix, 1/16 pie	270	N.A.	N.A.	10	90	N.A.
Weight Watchers, 1/2 pkg	160	1	2	4	35	5
Butter Brickle cake mix, Betty Crocker, 1/12 cake	250	2	4	10	90	55
no cholesterol recipe, 1/12 cake	220	2	2	6	50	0

*Less than 2% U.S. RDA
†All cakes, cupcakes, coffee cakes, and sweet rolls are frozen unless otherwise noted.

Sodium (mg)	Potassium (mg)	Protein (g)	Carbohy-drate (g)	Calcium (% U.S. RDA)	Iron (% U.S. RDA)	Vitamin A (% U.S. RDA)	Vitamin C (% U.S. RDA)
170	60	3	30	4	*	*	*
290	55	3	34	6	*	*	*
280	45	3	36	6	4	*	*
280	50	3	36	6	4	*	*
105	N.A.	2	37	6	*	*	*
190	50	2	33	4	4	*	*
200	50	2	33	4	4	*	*
290	80	3	36	4	4	2	*
160	N.A.	1	28	*	4	2	*
310	85	3	38	4	6	*	*
100	N.A.	2	28	2	8	6	*
280	280	4	32	4	6	*	4
390	110	4	50	15	4	2	*
125	N.A.	4	34	6	10	4	*
310	70	3	43	6	4	*	*
260	120	3	34	6	4	*	*
280	40	3	38	6	6	*	*
280	45	3	38	6	6	*	*

～ CAKES†

	Calories	Saturated fat (g)	Polyunsaturated fat (g)	Total fat (g)	Calories from fat	Cholesterol (mg)
Butter pecan cake mix, Betty Crocker, 1/12 cake	250	3	4	11	100	55
no cholesterol recipe, 1/12 cake	220	2	2	7	60	0
Carrot cake						
cake mix, 1/12 cake, all varieties	260	3	4	11	100	65
no cholesterol recipe, 1/12 cake	210	2	2	6	50	0
Pepperidge Farm, 1⅜ oz	140	N.A.	N.A.	8	70	N.A.
Sara Lee, iced single layer, 1/8 cake	250	N.A.	N.A.	13	120	25
Lights, 1 cake	170	N.A.	N.A.	4	35	5
snack cake, 1 cake	200	N.A.	N.A.	11	100	N.A.
Weight Watchers, 1/2 pkg	170	<1	2	5	45	5
Cheesecake						
Jell-O No Bake mix, 1/8 cake, all varieties	280	N.A.	N.A.	13	120	28
Pepperidge Farm American Collection, Manhattan Strawberry, 1 pkg	300	N.A.	N.A.	9	80	N.A.
Sara Lee, original, 1/6 cake, all varieties	230	N.A.	N.A.	9	80	N.A.
Classic snack cake, 1 cake	200	N.A.	N.A.	14	130	N.A.
Classics, 1/8 cake, French, strawberry French	250	N.A.	N.A.	15	140	20
Free & Light strawberry yogurt dessert, 1/10 cake	120	N.A.	N.A.	1	10	0
Lights, 1 cake, French, strawberry French	150	N.A.	N.A.	3	25	10
Weight Watchers, 1/2 pkg, all varieties	200	2	1	6	50	20
cheesecake mousse mix, 1/2 cup	60	N.A.	N.A.	2	18	N.A.

*Less than 2% U.S. RDA
†All cakes, cupcakes, coffee cakes, and sweet rolls are frozen unless otherwise noted.

Sodium (mg)	Potassium (mg)	Protein (g)	Carbohydrate (g)	Calcium (% U.S. RDA)	Iron (% U.S. RDA)	Vitamin A (% U.S. RDA)	Vitamin C (% U.S. RDA)
320	45	3	35	8	4	*	*
320	50	3	35	8	4	*	*
310	70	3	35	4	4	25	*
300	70	3	35	6	6	25	*
150	N.A.	1	17	*	2	15	2
240	N.A.	3	30	*	4	40	*
75	N.A.	4	30	6	6	30	*
190	N.A.	2	22	2	2	15	*
280	220	4	27	6	4	45	15
390	210	5	37	15	*	8	*
250	N.A.	6	49	6	4	*	2
170	N.A.	4	32	4	2	6	8
150	N.A.	4	16	2	*	10	*
125	N.A.	4	26	4	4	6	2
90	N.A.	2	26	4	4	8	4
80	N.A.	4	27	8	4	8	2
270	180	9	29	10	4	2	2
75	N.A.	4	12	20	*	2	*

~ CAKES†

	Calories	Saturated fat (g)	Polyunsaturated fat (g)	Total fat (g)	Calories from fat	Cholesterol (mg)
Cherry cake						
Betty Crocker mix, cherry chip, 1/12 cake	190	1	0	3	25	0
Duncan Hines Tierra Dessert mix, cherries and cream, 1/12 pkg	250	N.A.	N.A.	11	100	N.A.
Pepperidge Farm Dessert Light, 1 pkg	170	0	0	2	18	80
Weight Watchers cherries and cream, 1/2 pkg	190	1	3	6	50	5
Chocolate and devil's food cake						
cake mix, 1/12 cake, all varieties	260	4	4	13	120	61
no cholesterol recipe, 1/12 cake	240	2	2	10	90	0
Betty Crocker microwave mix, with frosting, 1/6 cake, all varieties	310	5	6	17	150	35
no cholesterol recipe, devil's food, 1/6 cake	240	3	2	9	80	0
pudding cake mix, 1/6 cake	230	N.A.	N.A.	5	45	N.A.
Duncan Hines mix, DeLights, 1/12 cake	180	2	1	5	25	35
Pepperidge Farm, devil's food, fudge layer, 1⅝ oz	180	N.A.	N.A.	10	90	N.A.
Dessert Light, mousse cake, 1 pkg	190	3	2	9	80	5
Pillsbury bundt mix, 1/16 cake, macaroon, tunnel of fudge	250	N.A.	N.A.	11	100	N.A.
microwave mix, 1/8 cake	210	N.A.	N.A.	13	120	N.A.
with frosting, 1/8 cake	300	N.A.	N.A.	17	150	N.A.
supreme mix, 1/8 cake	330	N.A.	N.A.	19	170	N.A.

*Less than 2% U.S. RDA
†All cakes, cupcakes, coffee cakes, and sweet rolls are frozen unless otherwise noted.

Sodium (mg)	Potassium (mg)	Protein (g)	Carbohy-drate (g)	Calcium (% U.S. RDA)	Iron (% U.S. RDA)	Vitamin A (% U.S. RDA)	Vitamin C (% U.S. RDA)
270	35	3	37	*	4	*	*
270	N.A.	4	34	10	2	*	*
35	N.A.	0	38	4	4	8	2
200	100	3	32	4	*	6	4
410	130	4	34	6	8	2	2
390	150	3	34	6	8	*	*
270	110	3	38	6	6	2	*
250	180	2	37	4	6	2	*
250	170	3	44	4	4	*	*
350	N.A.	3	32	6	4	*	*
140	N.A.	1	23	*	4	*	*
260	N.A.	3	25	2	6	*	*
310	105	3	37	*	6	*	*
260	70	2	23	4	4	*	*
310	90	2	36	4	4	*	*
340	140	3	39	6	6	*	*

～ CAKES†

	Calories	Saturated fat (g)	Polyunsaturated fat (g)	Total fat (g)	Calories from fat	Cholesterol (mg)
tunnel of fudge, ⅛ prepared cake	290	N.A.	N.A.	17	150	N.A.
Sara Lee, Free & Light, ⅛ cake	110	N.A.	N.A.	0	N.A.	0
Lights, 1 cake	150	N.A.	N.A.	5	45	10
snack cake, 1 cake	190	N.A.	N.A.	10	90	N.A.
three-layer cake, ⅛ cake	220	N.A.	N.A.	11	100	20
Weight Watchers, ½ pkg, chocolate, double fudge	190	<1	2	5	45	5
Chocolate-chip cake mix, 1/12 cake, all varieties	260	3	4	13	120	52
no cholesterol recipe, 1/12 cake	210	2	1	6	50	0
Cinnamon pecan streusel, Betty Crocker microwave mix, ⅙ cake	290	3	4	13	120	45
no cholesterol recipe	240	2	1	8	70	0
Coconut layer cake, Pepperidge Farm, 1⅝ oz	180	N.A.	N.A.	8	70	N.A.
Coffee cakes						
Drake, packaged, 1 cake	140	1	2	6	50	10
Entenmann's, packaged, no fat, 1 serving, all varieties	90	0	0	0	0	0
Freihofer's, packaged, low-fat, 1 serving, all varieties	90	1	1	2	18	0
Hostess, packaged, crumb, 1 cake	140	2	1	5	45	10
Lights, cinnamon, 1 cake	80	N.A.	N.A.	1	10	0
Pillsbury mix, apple cinnamon, ⅛ cake	240	N.A.	N.A.	7	60	N.A.
Pepperidge Farm American Collection, Amherst Apple Crumb, 1 pkg	260	N.A.	N.A.	13	120	N.A.
Sara Lee all butter, ⅛ cake, all varieties	180	N.A.	N.A.	9	80	N.A.

*Less than 2% U.S. RDA
†All cakes, cupcakes, coffee cakes, and sweet rolls are frozen unless otherwise noted.

Sodium (mg)	Potassium (mg)	Protein (g)	Carbohy-drate (g)	Calcium (% U.S. RDA)	Iron (% U.S. RDA)	Vitamin A (% U.S. RDA)	Vitamin C (% U.S. RDA)
320	135	3	36	6	6	*	*
140	N.A.	2	26	*	8	2	*
85	N.A.	4	23	8	8	6	*
125	N.A.	2	24	*	6	*	*
130	N.A.	3	26	2	8	*	*
220	180	5	33	8	6	*	6
320	70	3	35	6	6	*	*
300	55	3	36	8	4	*	*
210	45	3	39	6	4	*	*
220	45	3	39	6	4	*	*
120	N.A.	1	24	2	2	*	*
90	N.A.	2	18	2	4	*	*
90	N.A.	2	19	N.A.	N.A.	N.A.	N.A.
100	N.A.	1	16	N.A.	N.A.	N.A.	N.A.
90	N.A.	2	21	2	4	*	*
115	N.A.	1	19	2	2	*	*
150	75	3	40	4	6	*	*
180	N.A.	2	35	6	2	*	*
190	N.A.	3	21	*	6	4	*

CAKES†

	Calories	Saturated fat (g)	Polyunsaturated fat (g)	Total fat (g)	Calories from fat	Cholesterol (mg)
individual wrap, all varieties	270	N.A.	N.A.	14	130	N.A.
Weight Watchers with cinnamon streusel, ½ pkg	190	1	1	7	60	5
Cupcakes						
Duncan Hines, microwave Duncan Cups mix, 1 cake, all varieties	180	N.A.	N.A.	7	60	0
Entenmann's, packaged no fat, 1 cake	190	0	0	0	0	0
Hostess, packaged, creme filled, 1 cake	180	3	1	6	50	5
Dessert Cup, 1 cake	60	0	0	0	0	9
Lights, 1 cake, all flavors	130	N.A.	N.A.	1	10	0
Danish						
Hostess, packaged Sweet Good, 3¾ oz, apple, raspberry	400	10	1	21	190	20
Sara Lee individual, 1 danish, all varieties	130	N.A.	N.A.	7	60	N.A.
Danish twist, 1 danish, all varieties	200	N.A.	N.A.	10	90	13
Free & Light, apple, 1 danish	130	0	0	0	0	0
Doughnuts‡						
cake type						
Dunkin' Donuts, plain, glazed	300	N.A.	N.A.	18	160	7
Hostess, Donettes (½ oz), all varieties	60	2	1	3	25	5
family pack (1 oz)	120	3	1	6	50	5
pantry assortment (1⅔ oz)	190	5	1	10	90	10
Tastykake (1⅔ oz)	170	1	4	5	45	11

*Less than 2% U.S. RDA
†All cakes, cupcakes, coffee cakes, and sweet rolls are frozen unless otherwise noted.
‡Values for each doughnut listing are for 1 doughnut.

Sodium (mg)	Potassium (mg)	Protein (g)	Carbohy-drate (g)	Calcium (% U.S. RDA)	Iron (% U.S. RDA)	Vitamin A (% U.S. RDA)	Vitamin C (% U.S. RDA)
270	N.A.	4	32	2	6	4	8
250	80	3	28	2	4	*	*
140	N.A.	1	30	4	4	*	*
115	N.A.	2	48	N.A.	N.A.	N.A.	N.A.
290	80	2	30	10	6	*	*
120	N.A.	1	14	2	2	*	*
150	N.A.	2	28	*	4	*	*
320	120	4	48	10	8	*	*
130	N.A.	2	15	*	4	*	2
230	N.A.	3	23	*	6	*	4
120	N.A.	2	30	*	8	*	10
370	N.A.	4	34	N.A.	N.A.	N.A.	N.A.
70	30	1	7	*	2	*	*
150	40	2	14	*	4	*	*
250	65	3	23	2	6	*	*
240	N.A.	3	29	*	4	*	*

∼ CAKES†

	Calories	Saturated fat (g)	Polyunsaturated fat (g)	Total fat (g)	Calories from fat	Cholesterol (mg)
filled type, Dunkin' Donuts, all varieties	240	N.A.	N.A.	10	90	0
French cruller, Dunkin' Donuts	140	N.A.	N.A.	8	70	30
raised ring, glazed, Dunkin' Donuts	200	N.A.	N.A.	9	80	0
Frosting						
fluffy white mix, ¹⁄₁₂ mix	70	0	0	0	0	0
mix, ¹⁄₁₂ pkg, all varieties	160	2	2	8	70	0
ready-to-spread, ¹⁄₁₂ container, all varieties	150	3	<1	7	60	0
Gingerbread cake or dessert mix, 1/9 cake	210	2	<1	6	50	30
Lemon cake						
cake mix, ¹⁄₁₂ cake	260	3	5	11	100	60
no cholesterol recipe, ¹⁄₁₂ cake	240	2	3	9	80	0
Betty Crocker, chiffon mix, ¹⁄₁₂ cake	200	N.A.	N.A.	5	45	N.A.
pudding cake mix, ¹⁄₆ cake	230	N.A.	N.A.	5	45	N.A.
Pepperidge Farm, Lemon coconut, ¼ cake	280	N.A.	N.A.	13	120	N.A.
Dessert Light, 1 pkg	170	N.A.	N.A.	5	45	N.A.
Pillsbury bundt mix, tunnel of lemon, ¹⁄₁₆ cake	270	N.A.	N.A.	9	80	N.A.
microwave mix, ¹⁄₈ cake	220	N.A.	N.A.	13	120	N.A.
with frosting, ¹⁄₈ cake	300	N.A.	N.A.	17	150	N.A.
Sara Lee Lights, lemon cream cake, 1 pkg	180	N.A.	N.A.	6	50	10
Marble cake						
cake mix, ¹⁄₁₂ cake	260	3	4	11	100	63
no cholesterol recipe, ¹⁄₁₂ cake	220	2	2	7	60	0

*Less than 2% U.S. RDA
†All cakes, cupcakes, coffee cakes, and sweet rolls are frozen unless otherwise noted.

Sodium (mg)	Potassium (mg)	Protein (g)	Carbohydrate (g)	Calcium (% U.S. RDA)	Iron (% U.S. RDA)	Vitamin A (% U.S. RDA)	Vitamin C (% U.S. RDA)
260	N.A.	4	32	N.A.	N.A.	N.A.	N.A.
130	N.A.	2	16	N.A.	N.A.	N.A.	N.A.
230	N.A.	4	26	N.A.	N.A.	N.A.	N.A.
55	15	<1	16	*	*	*	*
85	60	<1	22	*	2	*	*
80	85	<1	24	*	*	*	*
320	160	3	36	4	10	*	*
290	30	3	36	6	6	*	*
290	25	3	36	8	6	*	*
200	60	4	36	2	4	*	*
270	35	2	45	4	2	*	*
220	N.A.	3	38	2	4	*	4
100	N.A.	4	26	4	2	2	*
300	90	2	45	6	4	*	*
180	20	2	23	6	2	*	*
220	35	2	37	6	2	*	*
60	N.A.	3	29	2	4	2	*
290	60	3	36	6	6	*	*
270	60	3	36	6	4	*	*

~ CAKES†

	Calories	Saturated fat (g)	Polyunsat- urated fat (g)	Total fat (g)	Calories from fat	Choles- terol (mg)
Peach Melba Shortcake, Charleston, Pepperidge Farm American Collection, 1 pkg	220	N.A.	N.A.	5	45	N.A.
Pineapple cake						
Betty Crocker upside down mix, 1/9 cake	250	4	<1	10	90	40
Duncan Hines mix, 1/12 cake	260	3	5	11	100	65
Pepperidge Farm, 1/12 cake	190	N.A.	N.A.	7	60	N.A.
Pillsbury bundt mix, 1/16 cake	260	N.A.	N.A.	9	80	N.A.
Pound cake						
Betty Crocker mix, 1/12 cake	200	3	1	9	80	35
Entenmann's, packaged no fat, 1 oz slice	70	0	0	0	0	0
Sara Lee, all butter, 1/10 cake	130	N.A.	N.A.	7	60	N.A.
Free & Light, 1/10 cake	70	0	0	0	0	0
snack cake, 1 cake	200	<1	<1	11	100	1
Rainbow Chip Cake Mix, Betty Crocker, 1/12 cake	250	3	4	11	100	55
Snack cakes, packaged						
Drake, Funny Bones, 1 cake	150	2	1	8	70	0
Ring Dings, 1 cake	180	3	1	10	90	0
Yankee Doodles, 1 cake	100	1	1	4	35	0
Yodels, 1 cake	150	2	1	9	80	5
Hostess, Ding Dongs, 1 cake	170	N.A.	N.A.	9	80	6
Ho Hos, 1 cake	120	N.A.	N.A.	6	50	8
King Dons, 1 cake	170	N.A.	N.A.	9	80	6
Sno Balls, 1 cake	140	N.A.	N.A.	2	18	2
Suzy Q's, 1 cake, banana, chocolate banana, chocolate	250	N.A.	N.A.	8	70	16
Twinkies, 1 cake	160	3	1	6	50	10
Lights, 1 cake	110	N.A.	N.A.	2	18	0

*Less than 2% U.S. RDA
†All cakes, cupcakes, coffee cakes, and sweet rolls are frozen unless otherwise noted.

Sodium (mg)	Potassium (mg)	Protein (g)	Carbohy-drate (g)	Calcium (% U.S. RDA)	Iron (% U.S. RDA)	Vitamin A (% U.S. RDA)	Vitamin C (% U.S. RDA)
170	N.A.	2	41	2	4	*	*
210	70	2	39	4	6	2	*
290	N.A.	3	36	6	6	*	*
130	N.A.	2	28	2	4	*	*
300	45	2	41	6	4	*	*
170	25	2	28	2	4	*	*
110	N.A.	2	16	N.A.	N.A.	N.A.	N.A.
85	N.A.	2	14	*	4	4	*
130	N.A.	1	16	*	4	4	*
190	N.A.	2	23	*	2	6	*
320	40	3	34	10	6	*	*
110	N.A.	3	18	2	2	*	*
115	N.A.	2	23	*	6	*	*
110	N.A.	1	16	*	2	*	*
65	N.A.	2	16	*	4	*	*
130	N.A.	1	21	2	8	*	*
70	N.A.	1	17	2	4	*	*
130	N.A.	1	21	2	8	*	*
90	N.A.	1	14	2	2	*	*
250	N.A.	2	43	4	6	*	*
180	N.A.	1	26	2	4	*	*
160	N.A.	2	21	2	4	*	*

~ CAKES†

	Calories	Saturated fat (g)	Polyunsaturated fat (g)	Total fat (g)	Calories from fat	Cholesterol (mg)
Nabisco, devil's food, 1 cake	70	<1	<1	1	10	0
marshmallow puffs fudge cakes, 1 cake	90	3	<1	4	35	0
marshmallow twirls fudge cakes, 1 cake	140	4	<1	6	50	0
Spice cake						
cake mix, ¹⁄₁₂ cake	260	3	5	11	100	60
no cholesterol recipe, ¹⁄₁₂ cake	240	2	3	9	80	0
Strawberry cake						
cake mix, ¹⁄₁₂ cake	260	3	5	12	110	68
no cholesterol recipe, ¹⁄₁₂ cake	220	2	2	7	60	0
Pepperidge Farm strawberry cream, ¹⁄₁₂ cake	190	N.A.	N.A.	7	60	N.A.
Strawberry shortcake						
Pepperidge Farm Dessert Light, 1 pkg	170	1	1	5	45	70
Sara Lee two-layer, ¹⁄₈ cake	190	N.A.	N.A.	8	70	N.A.
Streusel Swirl cake mix, Pillsbury, ¹⁄₁₆ cake, lemon, cinnamon	270	N.A.	N.A.	11	100	N.A.
microwave, ¹⁄₈ prepared cake	240	N.A.	N.A.	11	100	N.A.
Sweet rolls						
Hostess packaged honey buns, 1 bun, glazed or iced	400	10	1	22	200	18
Sweet Good Swirls, 1 bun, orange, pecan orange, pecan-caramel	290	7	2	14	130	10
Sara Lee Cinnamon Roll, 1 roll	230	N.A.	N.A.	11	100	N.A.
icing packet, ¼ packet	50	0	0	0	0	N.A.

*Less than 2% U.S. RDA
†All cakes, cupcakes, coffee cakes, and sweet rolls are frozen unless otherwise noted.

Sodium (mg)	Potassium (mg)	Protein (g)	Carbohy-drate (g)	Calcium (% U.S. RDA)	Iron (% U.S. RDA)	Vitamin A (% U.S. RDA)	Vitamin C (% U.S. RDA)
40	N.A.	1	15	*	2	*	*
45	N.A.	1	14	*	2	*	*
70	N.A.	1	20	*	4	*	*
310	50	3	36	8	6	*	*
310	55	3	36	8	6	*	*
290	30	3	36	6	6	*	*
290	30	3	36	6	4	*	*
120	N.A.	1	30	2	4	*	*
50	N.A.	2	30	4	4	4	20
90	N.A.	2	26	2	4	2	6
270	45	3	39	6	6	2	*
180	35	2	33	6	2	*	*
240	100	5	47	15	10	*	*
160	60	3	25	6	6	*	*
220	N.A.	3	31	*	2	4	*
0	N.A.	0	12	*	*	*	*

~ CAKES†/ COOKIES‡	Calories	Saturated fat (g)	Polyunsat- urated fat (g)	Total fat (g)	Calories from fat	Choles- terol (mg)
Weight Watchers, ½ pkg, all varieties	170	<1	<1	4	35	13
Vanilla cake						
cake mix, ¹⁄₁₂ cake	270	3	6	13	120	60
no cholesterol recipe, ¹⁄₁₂ cake	240	2	3	9	80	0
Betty Crocker microwave mix, rainbow chip frosting, ⅙ cake	320	5	6	17	150	35
Pepperidge Farm layer cake, 1⅝ oz	190	N.A.	N.A.	8	70	N.A.
White cake						
cake mix, ¹⁄₁₂ cake	240	2	4	10	90	33
no cholesterol recipe, ¹⁄₁₂ cake	220	2	2	7	60	0
Betty Crocker sour cream mix, ¹⁄₁₂ cake	180	1	0	3	25	0
Yellow cake						
cake mix, ¹⁄₁₂ cake	260	3	4	12	110	63
no cholesterol recipe, ¹⁄₁₂ cake	220	2	2	7	60	0
Duncan Hines mix, DeLights, ¹⁄₁₂ cake	180	1	1	4	35	35
Pepperidge Farm, golden layer cake, 1⅝ oz	180	N.A.	N.A.	9	60	N.A.
Pillsbury microwave mix, ⅛ cake	220	N.A.	N.A.	13	120	N.A.
with frosting	300	N.A.	N.A.	17	150	N.A.
Almond Toast, Stella D'Oro, 1 piece	60	N.A.	N.A.	1	10	<1
Almost Home, Nabisco, 1 cookie, all varieties	70	<1	<1	3	25	1
Angel Bar, Stella D'Oro, 1 piece	80	N.A.	N.A.	5	45	<1

*Less than 2% U.S. RDA
†All cakes, cupcakes, coffee cakes, and sweet rolls are frozen unless otherwise noted.
‡Packaged unless otherwise noted.

Sodium (mg)	Potassium (mg)	Protein (g)	Carbohy-drate (g)	Calcium (% U.S. RDA)	Iron (% U.S. RDA)	Vitamin A (% U.S. RDA)	Vitamin C (% U.S. RDA)
135	70	4	29	4	2	2	6
280	35	3	36	6	6	*	*
280	40	3	36	6	6	*	*
230	40	2	40	6	4	2	*
120	N.A.	1	25	*	*	*	*
270	45	3	36	4	4	*	*
250	40	3	37	6	4	*	*
300	40	3	36	*	4	*	*
300	50	3	36	6	4	*	*
290	35	3	36	6	4	*	*
275	N.A.	3	34	6	4	*	*
110	N.A.	1	24	2	2	*	*
170	25	2	23	6	2	*	*
220	60	2	36	6	4	*	*
N.A.	N.A.	1	10	N.A.	N.A.	N.A.	N.A.
60	N.A.	1	9	*	2	*	*
N.A.	N.A.	1	7	N.A.	N.A.	N.A.	N.A.

～ COOKIES†

	Calories	Saturated fat (g)	Polyunsaturated fat (g)	Total fat (g)	Calories from fat	Cholesterol (mg)
Angel Wings, Stella D'Oro, 1 piece	70	N.A.	N.A.	5	45	N.A.
Angelica Goodies, Stella D'Oro, 1 piece	110	N.A.	N.A.	4	35	<1
Anginetti, Stella D'Oro, 1 piece	30	N.A.	N.A.	1	10	<1
Animal Crackers, Sunshine, 13 crackers	130	1	<1	4	35	0
Anisette Sponge or Toast, Stella D'Oro, 1 piece	50	N.A.	N.A.	1	10	<1
jumbo toast, 1 piece	110	N.A.	N.A.	1	10	<1
Arrowroot Biscuit, Nabisco, 1 biscuit	20	<1	<1	1	10	1
Baby Bear Cookies, Keebler, ½ oz (3 cookies)	70	<1	<1	2	18	0
Baker's Bonus, Nabisco, ½ oz (1 cookie)	80	1	<1	3	25	3
Baker's Own, Nabisco, ½ oz (1 cookie), all flavors	80	<1	<1	2	18	0
Barnum's Animal Crackers, Nabisco, ½ oz (5 cookies)	60	<1	<1	2	18	1
Bavarian Fingers, Sunshine, 1 oz (2 cookies)	140	2	<1	6	50	0
Biscos Sugar Wafers, Nabisco, ½ oz (4 wafers)	70	<1	<1	3	25	0
Biscos Waffle Cremes, Nabisco, ½ oz (2 cookies)	70	<1	<1	4	35	0
Breakfast Treats, Stella D'Oro, 1 piece	100	N.A.	N.A.	4	35	<1
Brown Edge Wafers, Nabisco, 2 wafers	60	<1	<1	2	18	<1
Brownies						
brownie mix, 1 2"x 2" brownie	150	2	3	6	50	12
Betty Crocker MicroRave mix, 1 2"x2" brownie	160	2	1	7	60	0

*Less than 2% U.S. RDA
†Packaged unless otherwise noted.

Sodium (mg)	Potassium (mg)	Protein (g)	Carbohydrate (g)	Calcium (% U.S. RDA)	Iron (% U.S. RDA)	Vitamin A (% U.S. RDA)	Vitamin C (% U.S. RDA)
N.A.	N.A.	1	7	N.A.	N.A.	N.A.	N.A.
N.A.	N.A.	2	16	N.A.	N.A.	N.A.	N.A.
N.A.	N.A.	1	5	N.A.	N.A.	N.A.	N.A.
160	N.A.	2	21	*	4	*	*
N.A.	N.A.	1	10	N.A.	N.A.	N.A.	N.A.
N.A.	N.A.	2	23	N.A.	N.A.	N.A.	N.A.
15	N.A.	0	3	*	*	*	*
55	15	1	10	*	2	*	*
65	N.A.	1	12	*	2	*	*
80	N.A.	<1	12	2	2	*	*
70	N.A.	1	11	*	2	*	*
105	N.A.	2	20	*	6	*	*
20	N.A.	<1	10	*	*	*	*
20	N.A.	<1	10	*	*	*	*
N.A.	N.A.	2	15	N.A.	N.A.	N.A.	N.A.
35	N.A.	<1	8	*	2	*	*
100	60	1	21	*	4	*	*
110	150	2	23	*	4	*	*

～ COOKIES†

	Calories	Saturated fat (g)	Polyunsaturated fat (g)	Total fat (g)	Calories from fat	Cholesterol (mg)
Duncan Hines gourmet mix, 1 2″x2″ brownie	220	N.A.	N.A.	10	90	N.A.
Pepperidge Farm American Collection, frozen, Malibu Hot Fudge Peanut Butter, 1 pkg	400	N.A.	N.A.	21	190	N.A.
Monterey Hot Fudge Chocolate Chunk, 1 pkg	480	N.A.	N.A.	26	230	N.A.
Newport Hot Fudge, 1 pkg	400	N.A.	N.A.	20	180	N.A.
Pillsbury ultimate flavors mix, 1 2″x2″ brownie	170	N.A.	N.A.	7	60	N.A.
Weight Watchers, frozen, 1 brownie	100	<1	1	3	25	5
Butter Flavored Cookies, Sunshine, 1 oz (4 cookies)	120	1	<1	5	45	3
Cameo Creme Sandwich, Nabisco, ½ oz (1 cookie)	70	1	<1	3	25	0
Castelets, Stella D'Oro, 1 piece, regular, chocolate	70	N.A.	N.A.	3	25	<1
Chinese Dessert Cookie, Stella D'Oro, 1 piece	170	N.A.	N.A.	9	80	<1
Chips Ahoy!, Nabisco, ½ oz (1 cookie), all varieties (mini cookies: ½ oz = 6 cookies)	70	1	<1	4	35	1
Chips Deluxe, Keebler, ½ oz (1 cookie), all varieties	80	1	<1	4	35	3
Chocolate chip						
cookie mix, 2 cookies (no cholesterol recipe contains 0 mg cholesterol)	130	3	1	6	50	15
Duncan Hines, 2 cookies	110	2	<1	5	45	0
Keebler soft batch, 1 cookie, all varieties	80	1	<1	4	35	0
Nestlé toll house, ready-to-bake, 2 cookies	150	N.A.	N.A.	7	60	N.A.

*Less than 2% U.S. RDA
†Packaged unless otherwise noted.

Sodium (mg)	Potassium (mg)	Protein (g)	Carbohydrate (g)	Calcium (% U.S. RDA)	Iron (% U.S. RDA)	Vitamin A (% U.S. RDA)	Vitamin C (% U.S. RDA)
130	N.A.	2	29	2	6	*	*
190	N.A.	7	45	4	6	*	*
200	N.A.	5	56	4	6	*	*
160	N.A.	4	50	4	6	*	*
105	70	2	25	*	4	*	*
150	110	3	16	2	6	*	*
150	N.A.	2	17	*	4	*	*
50	N.A.	1	10	*	2	*	*
N.A.	N.A.	1	10	N.A.	N.A.	N.A.	N.A.
N.A.	N.A.	2	20	N.A.	N.A.	N.A.	N.A.
45	N.A.	1	9	*	*	*	*
60	30	<1	10	*	2	*	*
95	75	1	18	*	4	*	*
95	N.A.	1	15	*	4	*	*
65	25	<1	10	*	2	*	*
115	65	1	20	*	*	*	*

~ COOKIES†

	Calories	Saturated fat (g)	Polyunsaturated fat (g)	Total fat (g)	Calories from fat	Cholesterol (mg)
Pillsbury, 1 cookie, all varieties	70	<1	<1	3	25	3
Chocolate Chip Snaps, Nabisco, ½ oz (3 cookies)	70	1	<1	2	18	1
Chocolate Fudge Cookies, Keebler, ½ oz (1 cookie)	80	1	1	4	35	0
Chocolate Grahams, Nabisco, ½ oz (1 cookie)	60	2	<1	3	25	1
Chocolate Snaps, Nabisco, ½ oz (4 snaps)	70	1	<1	2	18	1
Coconut Cookie, Stella D'Oro, 1 cookie, dietetic	50	N.A.	N.A.	2	18	N.A.
Coconut Macaroons, Stella D'Oro, 1 piece	60	N.A.	N.A.	3	25	<1
Como Delights, Stella D'Oro, 1 piece	150	N.A.	N.A.	7	60	1
Cookie, coffee shop, Dunkin' Donuts, 1 cookie	200	N.A.	N.A.	10	90	28
Cookie Break Vanilla Creme, Nabisco, ½ oz (1 cookie)	50	<1	<1	2	18	1
Cookies 'n Fudge, Nabisco, 1 cookie, all varieties	60	1	<1	3	25	0
Deep Night Fudge Cookies, Stella D'Oro, 1 piece	70	N.A.	N.A.	4	35	N.A.
Dutch Apple Bar, Stella D'Oro, 1 piece	110	N.A.	N.A.	3	25	<1
Egg Biscuit, Stella D'Oro, 1 biscuit, all varieties but Roman (dietetic contains <10 mg sodium)	40	N.A.	N.A.	1	10	N.A.
Roman Egg Biscuit, 1 piece	140	N.A.	N.A.	5	45	<1
E. L. Fudge Cookies, Keebler, 1 cookie, all varieties	60	<1	<1	3	25	3
Famous Chocolate Wafers, Nabisco, 2 wafers	60	<1	<1	2	18	<1
Fig Bars, Sunshine, 2 bars	100	<1	<1	2	18	1

*Less than 2% U.S. RDA
†Packaged unless otherwise noted.

Sodium (mg)	Potassium (mg)	Protein (g)	Carbohy-drate (g)	Calcium (% U.S. RDA)	Iron (% U.S. RDA)	Vitamin A (% U.S. RDA)	Vitamin C (% U.S. RDA)
45	25	1	9	*	*	*	*
50	N.A.	1	11	*	2	*	*
70	25	1	12	*	2	*	*
30	N.A.	1	7	*	2	*	*
75	N.A.	1	11	*	2	*	*
5	N.A.	1	6	N.A.	N.A.	N.A.	N.A.
N.A.	N.A.	1	7	N.A.	N.A.	N.A.	N.A.
N.A.	N.A.	2	18	N.A.	N.A.	N.A.	N.A.
105	N.A.	3	25	N.A.	N.A.	N.A.	N.A.
35	N.A.	1	7	*	*	*	*
45	N.A.	<1	7	*	*	*	*
N.A.	N.A.	N.A.	8	N.A.	N.A.	N.A.	N.A.
N.A.	N.A.	1	19	N.A.	N.A.	N.A.	N.A.
5	N.A.	2	7	N.A.	N.A.	N.A.	N.A.
N.A.	N.A.	3	20	N.A.	N.A.	N.A.	N.A.
45	20	<1	8	*	*	*	*
90	N.A.	<1	9	*	2	*	*
70	N.A.	1	20	*	4	*	*

~ COOKIES†

	Calories	Saturated fat (g)	Polyunsaturated fat (g)	Total fat (g)	Calories from fat	Cholesterol (mg)
Fig Newtons (see Newtons, below)						
Fig Pastry, dietetic, Stella D'Oro, 1 piece	90	N.A.	N.A.	4	35	N.A.
Fortune Cookies, La Choy, 1 cookie	16	N.A.	N.A.	<1	N.A.	0
French Vanilla Creme, Keebler, ½ oz (1 cookie)	80	<1	<1	4	35	0
Fruit Cookies, Pepperidge Farm, 1 cookie, strawberry, apricot-raspberry	50	1	0	2	18	5
Fruit Slices, Stella D'Oro, 1 piece, dietetic	60	N.A.	N.A.	2	18	<1
Fudge Family Bears, Sunshine, 2 cookies, all varieties	140	2	<1	6	50	0
Fudge Sticks, Keebler, ½ oz (2 cookies)	100	3	<1	5	45	0
Fudge Stripes, Keebler, ½ oz (1 cookie)	50	2	<1	3	25	0
Giggles Sandwich Cookie, Nabisco, ½ oz (1 cookie)	60	<1	<1	3	25	1
Ginger snaps						
Nabisco, Old Fashioned, ¼ oz (1 snap)	30	<1	<1	1	10	1
Sunshine, 5 snaps	100	1	<1	3	25	0
Golden Bars, Stella D'Oro, 1 piece	110	N.A.	N.A.	4	35	<1
Golden Fruit Raisin Biscuits, Sunshine, 1 oz (2 cookies)	150	1	<1	3	25	1
Graham Bites or Snacks, Nabisco, ½ oz (11 pieces), all varieties	60	<1	<1	2	18	0
Graham Cookies, Bugs Bunny, Nabisco, ½ oz (5 cookies)	60	<1	<1	2	18	0
Graham crackers, Nabisco, ½ oz (2 crackers)	60	<1	<1	1	10	0

*Less than 2% U.S. RDA
†Packaged unless otherwise noted.

Sodium (mg)	Potassium (mg)	Protein (g)	Carbohydrate (g)	Calcium (% U.S. RDA)	Iron (% U.S. RDA)	Vitamin A (% U.S. RDA)	Vitamin C (% U.S. RDA)
5	N.A.	2	13	N.A.	N.A.	N.A.	N.A.
0	0	<1	4	*	*	*	*
80	15	<1	12	*	2	*	*
25	N.A.	0	8	*	*	*	*
N.A.	N.A.	1	9	N.A.	N.A.	N.A.	N.A.
125	N.A.	2	18	*	6	*	*
35	35	<1	13	*	2	*	*
55	15	<1	7	*	*	*	*
20	N.A.	1	8	*	2	*	*
45	N.A.	<1	6	*	2	*	*
120	N.A.	1	16	*	4	*	*
N.A.	N.A.	2	16	N.A.	N.A.	N.A.	N.A.
80	N.A.	2	29	*	4	*	*
70	N.A.	1	11	*	2	*	*
70	N.A.	1	11	*	2	*	*
90	N.A.	1	11	*	2	*	*

~ COOKIES†

	Calories	Saturated fat (g)	Polyunsaturated fat (g)	Total fat (g)	Calories from fat	Cholesterol (mg)
Graham Crumbs, Nabisco, 1 oz (¼ cup)	120	N.A.	N.A.	2	18	N.A.
Grahamy Bears, Sunshine, 1 oz (9 cookies)	130	1	<1	5	45	0
Grasshopper Cookies, Keebler, ½ oz (2 cookies)	70	3	<1	3	25	0
Halvah, natural, Fantastic Foods, 1½ oz (1 bar)	230	N.A.	N.A.	10	90	N.A.
Heyday Bars, Nabisco, ¾ oz (1 bar), all varieties	110	2	1	6	50	0
Holiday Trinkets, Stella D'Oro, 1 piece	40	N.A.	N.A.	2	18	<1
Hostess or Lady Stella Assortment, Stella D'Oro, 1 piece	40	N.A.	N.A.	2	18	<1
Hydrox, Sunshine, 1 oz (3 cookies)	160	2	<1	7	60	0
Iced Animal Cookies, Keebler, ½ oz (3 cookies)	70	<1	<1	2	18	0
Ideal Bars, Nabisco, ¾ oz (1 bar), chocolate, peanut	90	2	<1	5	45	1
Imported Danish Cookies, Nabisco, ½ oz (2 cookies)	70	<1	<1	4	35	0
Kichel, Stella D'Oro, 1 piece, dietetic	8	N.A.	N.A.	<1	N.A.	N.A.
Kudos, Mars, 1.3 oz (1 bar)	190	N.A.	N.A.	12	110	N.A.
Lorna Doone, Nabisco, ½ oz (3 cookies)	70	<1	<1	4	35	4
Love Cookies, Stella D'Oro, 1 piece	110	N.A.	N.A.	5	45	<1
Magic Middles, Keebler, ½ oz (1 cookie), all flavors	80	1	1	5	45	3
Mallomars, Nabisco, ½ oz (1 cake)	60	1	<1	3	25	0
Mallopuffs, Sunshine, 1 oz (2 cookies)	130	2	<1	4	35	0

*Less than 2% U.S. RDA
†Packaged unless otherwise noted.

Sodium (mg)	Potassium (mg)	Protein (g)	Carbohy- drate (g)	Calcium (% U.S. RDA)	Iron (% U.S. RDA)	Vitamin A (% U.S. RDA)	Vitamin C (% U.S. RDA)
180	N.A.	2	22	*	4	*	*
160	N.A.	2	21	*	4	*	*
35	45	<1	10	*	2	*	*
N.A.	N.A.	8	17	N.A.	N.A.	N.A.	N.A.
60	N.A.	2	12	2	2	*	*
N.A.	N.A.	1	5	N.A.	N.A.	N.A.	N.A.
N.A.	N.A.	1	6	N.A.	N.A.	N.A.	N.A.
140	N.A.	2	21	*	6	*	*
65	20	1	12	*	2	*	*
80	N.A.	2	11	*	2	*	*
15	N.A.	1	9	*	2	*	*
5	N.A.	<1	<1	N.A.	N.A.	N.A.	N.A.
70	N.A.	4	18	2	2	*	*
65	N.A.	1	9	*	2	*	*
N.A.	N.A.	1	13	N.A.	N.A.	N.A.	N.A.
25	10	1	9	*	*	*	*
20	N.A.	1	9	*	2	*	*
75	N.A.	1	24	*	2	*	*

∿ COOKIES†

	Calories	Saturated fat (g)	Polyunsaturated fat (g)	Total fat (g)	Calories from fat	Cholesterol (mg)
Marguerite, Stella D'Oro, 1 piece, chocolate, vanilla	70	N.A.	N.A.	3	25	<1
Mini Middles, Keebler, ½ oz (4 cookies), all varieties	80	1	1	5	45	0
Molasses Cookies, Pantry, Nabisco, ½ oz (1 cookie)	80	<1	<1	3	25	0
Mystic Mint, Nabisco, ½ oz (1 cookie)	90	3	<1	5	45	1
Newtons, Nabisco, ½ oz (1 cookie), fig	60	<1	<1	1	10	1
apple, raspberry, strawberry, ¾ oz (1 cookie)	80	<1	<1	1	10	1
variety pack, 1 oz (1 cookie)	120	1	<1	3	25	1
Nilla Wafers, Nabisco, 3 wafers, regular, cinnamon	50	<1	<1	2	18	3
Nutter Butter, Nabisco, ½ oz (1 cookie)	70	<1	<1	3	25	1
peanut creme patties, ½ oz (2 cookies)	80	<1	<1	4	35	0
Oat cookies						
Duncan Hines, 2 cookies, oatmeal raisin	110	1	<1	5	45	0
from mix, 2 cookies, oatmeal raisin	130	N.A.	N.A.	6	50	N.A.
Entenmann's no-fat, 2 cookies, oatmeal raisin	80	0	0	0	0	0
Sunshine, 2 cookies, all varieties	120	1	<1	6	50	0
Oreo, Nabisco, regular, ½ oz (1 cookie)	50	<1	<1	2	18	1
Big Stuf, 1¾ oz (1 cookie)	250	4	1	12	110	3
Double Stuf, ½ oz (1 cookie)	70	1	<1	4	35	1
fudge covered, ¾ oz (1 cookie)	110	4	<1	6	50	1

*Less than 2% U.S. RDA
†Packaged unless otherwise noted.

Sodium (mg)	Potassium (mg)	Protein (g)	Carbohy-drate (g)	Calcium (% U.S. RDA)	Iron (% U.S. RDA)	Vitamin A (% U.S. RDA)	Vitamin C (% U.S. RDA)
N.A.	N.A.	1	10	N.A.	N.A.	N.A.	N.A.
35	40	1	10	*	4	*	*
75	N.A.	1	13	*	6	*	*
65	N.A.	1	11	*	2	*	*
60	N.A.	1	11	*	2	*	*
55	N.A.	1	15	*	2	*	*
110	N.A.	1	23	*	4	*	*
40	N.A.	<1	9	*	2	*	*
50	N.A.	1	9	*	2	*	*
45	N.A.	2	8	*	2	*	*
75	N.A.	1	15	2	4	*	*
70	N.A.	2	18	2	4	*	*
120	N.A.	1	17	*	*	*	*
110	N.A.	1	16	*	4	*	*
75	N.A.	1	8	*	2	*	*
220	N.A.	2	33	*	6	*	*
75	N.A.	1	9	*	2	*	*
80	N.A.	1	13	*	2	*	*

~ COOKIES†

	Calories	Saturated fat (g)	Polyunsaturated fat (g)	Total fat (g)	Calories from fat	Cholesterol (mg)
O.T. Bears Cookies, Sunshine, 1 oz (9 cookies)	130	1	<1	5	45	0
Peach-Apricot Pastry, Stella D'Oro, 1 piece (dietetic contains <10 mg sodium)	90	N.A.	N.A.	4	35	<1
Peanut butter cookie						
Duncan Hines mix, 2 cookies (no cholesterol recipe has 0 mg cholesterol)	140	1	2	7	60	15
Nutter Butter (see Nutter Butter, above)						
Pillsbury, 1 cookie	70	<1	<1	3	25	5
Pecan Sandies, Keebler, ½ oz (1 cookie)	80	1	<1	5	45	3
Pecan Shortbread, Nabisco, ½ oz (1 cookie)	80	1	<1	5	45	1
Pepperidge Farm Cookies						
American Collection, 1 cookie, all varieties	110	N.A.	N.A.	6	50	5
Distinctive Cookies, 3 cookies, all varieties	220	N.A.	N.A.	11	100	3
Old Fashioned Cookies, 3 cookies, all varieties	150	N.A.	N.A.	8	70	3
Special Collection, 2 cookies	140	N.A.	N.A.	8	70	N.A.
Pfeffernusse, Stella D'Oro, 1 piece	40	N.A.	N.A.	1	10	<1
Pinwheels, Nabisco, 1 cake	130	2	<1	5	45	0
Pitter Patter Cookies, Keebler, ½ oz (1 cookie)	90	<1	<1	4	35	0
Prune Pastry, Stella D'Oro, 1 piece, dietetic	90	N.A.	N.A.	4	35	N.A.
Pure Chocolate Middles, Nabisco, ½ oz (1 cookie)	80	2	<1	5	45	3
Raisin Bakes Fruit Bars, Health Valley, 1 bar	100	N.A.	N.A.	3	25	0

*Less than 2% U.S. RDA
†Packaged unless otherwise noted.

Sodium (mg)	Potassium (mg)	Protein (g)	Carbohy-drate (g)	Calcium (% U.S. RDA)	Iron (% U.S. RDA)	Vitamin A (% U.S. RDA)	Vitamin C (% U.S. RDA)
160	N.A.	2	21	*	4	*	*
N.A.	N.A.	1	14	N.A.	N.A.	N.A.	N.A.
120	N.A.	3	15	*	2	*	*
75	20	1	9	*	*	*	*
75	10	<1	9	*	2	*	*
40	N.A.	1	8	*	2	*	*
75	N.A.	1	15	*	*	*	*
95	N.A.	1	24	*	*	*	*
100	N.A.	1	19	*	*	*	*
55	N.A.	1	14	*	2	*	*
N.A.	N.A.	1	7	N.A.	N.A.	N.A.	N.A.
40	N.A.	1	20	*	4	*	*
115	40	2	12	*	2	*	*
5	N.A.	2	13	N.A.	N.A.	N.A.	N.A.
35	N.A.	1	9	2	2	*	*
20	105	2	16	*	20	*	*

~ COOKIES†/ GELATIN	Calories	Saturated fat (g)	Polyunsaturated fat (g)	Total fat (g)	Calories from fat	Cholesterol (mg)
Royal Nuggets, Stella D'Oro, 1 piece	2	N.A.	N.A.	<1	N.A.	<1
School House Cookies, Sunshine, 1 oz (15 cookies)	120	1	<1	4	35	0
Sesame Cookie, Stella D'Oro, 1 piece (dietetic contains <10 mg sodium)	50	N.A.	N.A.	2	18	<1
Social Tea Biscuits, Nabisco, ⅙ oz (1 biscuit)	20	<1	<1	1	10	1
Suddenly S'mores, Nabisco, ¾ oz (1 cookie)	100	2	<1	4	35	0
Sugar cookies						
Duncan Hines mix, 2 cookies	130	N.A.	N.A.	6	50	N.A.
Keebler soft batch, 1 cookie	80	1	<1	5	45	0
Pillsbury, 1 cookie	70	<1	<1	3	25	5
Sugar Wafers, Sunshine, 1 oz (3 wafers), all varieties	130	1	<1	6	50	1
Swiss Fudge Cookie, Stella D'Oro, 1 piece	70	N.A.	N.A.	3	25	<1
Teddy Grahams, Nabisco, ½ oz (11 pieces), all flavors	60	<1	<1	2	18	0
Bearwich's, ½ oz (4 cookies), all flavors	70	<1	<1	3	25	0
Uneeda Biscuits, Nabisco, ½ oz (3 biscuits)	60	<1	<1	2	18	0
Vanilla wafers						
Keebler, ½ oz (4 wafers)	80	1	<1	3	25	0
Sunshine, 1 oz (6 wafers)	130	2	<1	6	50	5
Vienna Fingers, Sunshine, 2 cookies	140	1	<1	6	50	0
dry, 1 packet	25	0	0	0	0	N.A.
D-Zerta Low Calorie, ½ cup, all flavors	8	0	0	0	0	0

*Less than 2% U.S. RDA
†Packaged unless otherwise noted.

Sodium (mg)	Potassium (mg)	Protein (g)	Carbohy-drate (g)	Calcium (% U.S. RDA)	Iron (% U.S. RDA)	Vitamin A (% U.S. RDA)	Vitamin C (% U.S. RDA)
N.A.	N.A.	<1	<1	N.A.	N.A.	N.A.	N.A.
100	N.A.	2	20	*	4	*	*
N.A.	N.A.	1	6	N.A.	N.A.	N.A.	N.A.
20	N.A.	<1	4	*	*	*	*
90	N.A.	1	15	*	2	*	*
70	N.A.	1	17	*	2	*	*
80	10	<1	10	*	*	*	*
70	5	1	9	*	*	*	*
40	N.A.	2	17	*	4	*	*
N.A.	N.A.	1	9	N.A.	N.A.	N.A.	N.A.
90	N.A.	1	11	*	2	*	*
65	N.A.	1	10	*	2	*	*
100	N.A.	1	10	*	4	*	*
60	20	<1	10	*	2	*	*
105	N.A.	1	18	*	2	*	*
125	N.A.	1	21	*	2	*	*
N.A.	N.A.	6	0	N.A.	N.A.	N.A.	N.A.
0	50	2	0	*	*	*	*

~ GELATIN/ MUFFINS†/ PIES & PASTRIES‡	Calories	Saturated fat (g)	Polyunsat- urated fat (g)	Total fat (g)	Calories from fat	Choles- terol (mg)
Jell-O, ½ cup, average values, all flavors	80	0	0	0	0	0
sugar-free	8	0	0	0	0	0
Jell-O 1-2-3, ⅔ cup	130	N.A.	N.A.	2	18	0
Ice Cream Products (see Dairy Products & Eggs)						
Regular mix, 12 muffins per pkg, all varieties	120	1	1	5	45	22
no cholesterol recipe	120	1	1	4	35	0
Duncan Hines bakery style mix, 12 per pkg, all varieties	200	N.A.	N.A.	8	70	N.A.
Dunkin' Donuts coffee shop style, all varieties	310	N.A.	N.A.	10	90	23
Frozen, 1 muffin, all varieties	210	N.A.	N.A.	7	60	N.A.
Sara Lee Free & Light, blueberry	120	0	0	0	0	0
Weight Watchers, ½ of 5-oz pkg, all varieties	170	1	1	5	45	10
Hostess, 1½ oz, oat bran, banana nut oat bran	160	1	4	7	60	0
2 oz, oatmeal goodness varieties	140	N.A.	N.A.	2	18	0
Mini Muffins, 2-oz pkg (5 muffins), all varieties	250	2	8	15	140	42
Apple crisp						
Pepperidge Farm American Collection, Berkshire Apple Crisp, 1 pkg	250	N.A.	N.A.	8	70	N.A.
Weight Watchers, ½ pkg	190	<1	1	5	45	N.A.
Apple Dumpling, Pepperidge Farm, 3 oz	260	N.A.	N.A.	13	120	N.A.
Apple Pastry, Stella D'Oro, 1 piece, dietetic	90	N.A.	N.A.	4	35	N.A.
Apple pie						

*Less than 2% U.S. RDA
†Values are for 1 muffin unless otherwise noted.
‡Frozen unless otherwise noted.

Sodium (mg)	Potassium (mg)	Protein (g)	Carbohy-drate (g)	Calcium (% U.S. RDA)	Iron (% U.S. RDA)	Vitamin A (% U.S. RDA)	Vitamin C (% U.S. RDA)
60	0	2	19	*	*	*	*
60	0	1	0	*	*	*	*
55	0	2	27	*	*	*	*
160	80	2	17	2	4	*	*
160	80	2	19	2	2	*	*
240	N.A.	2	30	*	4	*	*
450	N.A.	7	50	N.A.	N.A.	N.A.	N.A.
270	N.A.	4	34	6	10	10	2
140	N.A.	3	28	15	25	25	2
240	100	3	31	4	4	4	*
160	55	2	21	2	4	*	*
160	N.A.	5	26	8	10	*	*
170	70	3	28	2	4	*	*
130	N.A.	2	43	4	6	*	*
190	50	1	40	*	4	*	*
230	N.A.	2	33	*	4	*	2
5	N.A.	1	14	N.A.	N.A.	N.A.	N.A.

∿ PIES & PASTRIES†

	Calories	Saturated fat (g)	Polyunsaturated fat (g)	Total fat (g)	Calories from fat	Cholesterol (mg)
Banquet family size, ⅙ of 20-oz pie	250	N.A.	N.A.	11	100	N.A.
Hostess packaged snack pie, 1 pie	390	N.A.	N.A.	19	170	13
Mrs. Smith's, ⅛ of pie	370	4	3	20	180	0
Dutch apple, ⅛ of pie	380	3	3	16	140	0
pie in minutes, ⅛ of pie	210	2	2	9	80	0
Pepperidge Farm American Collection, Apple Berry Pie, 1 pkg	280	N.A.	N.A.	5	45	N.A.
Pet-Ritz, ⅙ of 26-oz pie	330	N.A.	N.A.	12	110	N.A.
Sara Lee homestyle, ⅒ of 9″ pie	280	N.A.	N.A.	12	110	0
country apple pie, 1 pie	230	N.A.	N.A.	9	80	N.A.
Free & Light, apple streusel, ⅛ pie	170	N.A.	N.A.	2	18	0
homestyle Dutch apple, ⅒ of 9″ pie	300	N.A.	N.A.	12	110	0
homestyle high pie, ⅒ of 10″ pie	400	N.A.	N.A.	23	210	0
Weight Watchers, ½ pkg	200	1	2	5	45	5
Apple turnover						
Pepperidge Farm, 1 pastry	300	N.A.	N.A.	17	150	N.A.
Pillsbury, 1 refrigerated turnover	170	3	<1	8	70	5
Banana cream pie						
Banquet, ⅙ of 14-oz pie	180	N.A.	N.A.	10	90	N.A.
Jell-O No Bake mix, ⅛ pie	240	N.A.	N.A.	14	130	30
Pet-Ritz, ⅙ of 14-oz pie	170	N.A.	N.A.	9	80	N.A.
Blackberry pie						
Banquet family size, ⅙ of 20-oz pie	270	N.A.	N.A.	11	100	N.A.
Hostess packaged snack pie, 1 pie	380	N.A.	N.A.	15	140	15

*Less than 2% U.S. RDA
†Frozen unless otherwise noted.

Sodium (mg)	Potassium (mg)	Protein (g)	Carbohy-drate (g)	Calcium (% U.S. RDA)	Iron (% U.S. RDA)	Vitamin A (% U.S. RDA)	Vitamin C (% U.S. RDA)
290	N.A.	2	37	*	6	*	6
490	N.A.	4	56	4	8	*	*
350	80	2	45	*	*	2	N.A.
250	100	2	56	*	*	2	N.A.
250	N.A.	2	29	*	*	*	*
150	N.A.	2	57	4	6	*	*
390	130	2	53	2	6	*	6
220	N.A.	2	42	*	6	*	2
250	N.A.	2	36	*	6	4	2
140	N.A.	1	36	2	4	2	2
310	N.A.	2	45	*	4	*	2
450	N.A.	3	46	*	6	*	2
280	80	2	39	2	6	*	2
210	N.A.	3	34	*	4	*	4
320	30	2	23	*	2	*	*
150	N.A.	2	21	4	6	*	*
300	95	3	27	6	*	8	*
160	60	2	22	2	6	*	*
350	N.A.	3	40	2	6	*	8
360	N.A.	4	55	6	10	*	*

∾ PIES & PASTRIES†	Calories	Saturated fat (g)	Polyunsaturated fat (g)	Total fat (g)	Calories from fat	Cholesterol (mg)
Blueberry pie						
Banquet family size, ⅙ of 20-oz pie	270	N.A.	N.A.	11	100	N.A.
Hostess packaged snack pie, 1 pie	410	N.A.	N.A.	17	150	1
Mrs. Smith's, ⅛ of 9" pie	350	3	3	16	140	0
pie in minutes, ⅛ of pie	220	2	2	9	80	0
Pet-Ritz, ⅙ of 26-oz pie	370	N.A.	N.A.	12	110	N.A.
Sara Lee homestyle, ⅒ of 9" pie	300	N.A.	N.A.	12	110	0
Blueberry turnover, Pepperidge Farm, 1 pastry	320	N.A.	N.A.	19	170	N.A.
Boston cream pie (see Cakes, above)						
Cherry pie						
Banquet family size, ⅙ of 20-oz pie	250	N.A.	N.A.	11	100	N.A.
Hostess packaged snack pie, 1 pie	460	9	1	20	180	15
Mrs. Smith's, ⅛ of 9" pie	350	3	3	16	140	0
pie in minutes, ⅛ of pie	220	2	2	9	80	0
Pet-Ritz, ⅙ of 26-oz pie	300	N.A.	N.A.	12	110	N.A.
Sara Lee homestyle, ⅒ of 9" pie	270	N.A.	N.A.	13	120	0
Free & Light, cherry streusel, ⅒ of pie	160	N.A.	N.A.	2	18	0
Cherry turnover						
Pepperidge Farm, 1 pastry	310	N.A.	N.A.	19	170	N.A.
Pillsbury, 1 refrigerated turnover	170	3	<1	8	70	5
Chocolate pie						
Banquet chocolate cream, ⅙ of 14-oz pie	190	N.A.	N.A.	10	90	N.A.
Hostess packaged pudding snack pie, 1 pie	490	N.A.	N.A.	19	170	21

*Less than 2% U.S. RDA
†Frozen unless otherwise noted.

Sodium (mg)	Potassium (mg)	Protein (g)	Carbohy- drate (g)	Calcium (% U.S. RDA)	Iron (% U.S. RDA)	Vitamin A (% U.S. RDA)	Vitamin C (% U.S. RDA)
350	N.A.	3	40	*	6	*	6
450	N.A.	5	60	8	10	*	*
300	70	2	49	*	*	*	N.A.
240	N.A.	2	32	*	*	*	*
330	105	3	50	2	6	*	6
210	N.A.	2	45	*	10	*	*
240	N.A.	3	32	*	4	*	10
260	N.A.	3	36	*	6	4	4
380	125	4	65	8	10	*	2
300	130	2	49	*	*	4	N.A.
200	N.A.	2	32	*	*	*	*
330	150	3	48	2	6	8	4
270	N.A.	2	37	*	6	2	*
140	N.A.	2	34	2	6	2	*
290	N.A.	3	32	*	4	*	8
310	30	2	24	*	2	*	6
110	N.A.	2	24	4	6	*	*
440	N.A.	5	76	10	10	*	*

~ PIES & PASTRIES†

	Calories	Saturated fat (g)	Polyunsaturated fat (g)	Total fat (g)	Calories from fat	Cholesterol (mg)
Jell-O No Bake mix, chocolate mousse, ⅛ of pie	260	N.A.	N.A.	17	150	30
Pet-Ritz chocolate cream, ⅙ of 14-oz pie	190	N.A.	N.A.	8	70	N.A.
Weight Watchers chocolate mocha, ½ pkg	160	3	<1	5	45	5
Coconut cream pie						
Banquet, ⅙ of 14-oz pie	190	N.A.	N.A.	11	100	N.A.
Jell-O No Bake mix, ⅛ of pie	260	N.A.	N.A.	16	140	30
Pet-Ritz, ⅙ of 14-oz pie	190	N.A.	N.A.	8	70	N.A.
Eclair, chocolate with custard filling	240	4	N.A.	14	130	N.A.
Egg custard pie, Pet-Ritz, ⅙ of 24-oz pie	200	N.A.	N.A.	8	70	N.A.
Fruit pies, Drake packaged, 1 pie, all varieties	220	2	1	10	90	0
Fruit Squares, Pepperidge Farm, 1 pastry, all varieties	230	N.A.	N.A.	12	110	N.A.
Fudge brownie pie, Sara Lee snack cake, 1 pie	280	N.A.	N.A.	14	130	N.A.
Lemon pie						
Banquet lemon creme, ⅙ of 14-oz pie	170	N.A.	N.A.	9	80	N.A.
Hostess packaged snack pie, 1 pie	400	N.A.	N.A.	20	180	19
Mrs. Smith's lemon meringue, ⅛ of 8″ pie	210	1	1	5	45	30
Pet-Ritz lemon cream, ⅙ of 14-oz pie	190	N.A.	N.A.	9	80	N.A.
Mincemeat, None Such, ready-to-use, ⅓ cup	210	N.A.	N.A.	1	10	N.A.
Mincemeat pie						
Banquet family size, ⅙ of 20-oz pie	260	N.A.	N.A.	11	100	N.A.

*Less than 2% U.S. RDA
†Frozen unless otherwise noted.

Sodium (mg)	Potassium (mg)	Protein (g)	Carbohy-drate (g)	Calcium (% U.S. RDA)	Iron (% U.S. RDA)	Vitamin A (% U.S. RDA)	Vitamin C (% U.S. RDA)
430	240	4	25	8	4	8	*
150	80	1	27	2	6	*	*
150	180	5	23	8	2	*	*
120	N.A.	2	22	4	6	*	*
300	115	3	27	6	*	8	*
150	45	2	27	2	6	*	*
80	120	6	23	8	4	6	*
N.A.	N.A.	5	28	8	4	4	*
135	N.A.	2	30	*	6	*	*
180	N.A.	2	28	*	6	*	6
170	N.A.	4	35	2	8	4	*
120	N.A.	2	23	4	6	*	4
430	N.A.	4	58	10	8	*	*
130	80	2	38	*	*	*	*
150	50	2	26	2	6	*	*
260	80	1	49	2	4	*	*
370	N.A.	3	38	*	6	*	*

～ PIES & PASTRIES†

	Calories	Saturated fat (g)	Polyunsaturated fat (g)	Total fat (g)	Calories from fat	Cholesterol (mg)
Pet-Ritz, ⅙ of 26-oz pie	280	N.A.	N.A.	9	80	N.A.
Sara Lee homestyle, ⅒ of 9″ pie	300	N.A.	N.A.	13	120	0
Mississippi mud pie, Pepperidge Farm American Collection, 1 pkg	410	N.A.	N.A.	30	270	N.A.
Peach pie						
Banquet family size, ⅙ of 20-oz pie	245	N.A.	N.A.	11	100	N.A.
Hostess packaged snack pie, 1 pie	380	N.A.	N.A.	15	140	13
Mrs. Smith's, ⅛ of 9″ pie	330	3	2	15	140	0
pie in minutes, ⅛ of pie	210	2	2	9	80	0
Pet-Ritz, ⅙ of 26-oz pie	320	N.A.	N.A.	12	110	N.A.
Sara Lee homestyle, ⅒ of 9″ pie	280	N.A.	N.A.	12	110	0
Peach turnover, Pepperidge Farm, 1 pastry	320	N.A.	N.A.	19	170	N.A.
Pecan pie						
Mrs. Smith's pie in minutes, ⅛ of pie	330	2	4	13	120	35
Sara Lee homestyle, ⅒ of 9″ pie	400	N.A.	N.A.	18	160	55
Southern pecan pie, 1 snack pie	260	N.A.	N.A.	13	120	N.A.
Pie crust						
Betty Crocker mix, ⅟₁₆ pkg or ⅛ stick	120	2	<1	8	70	0
Pet-Ritz frozen shells, ⅙ regular shell	110	N.A.	N.A.	7	60	7
⅙ deep dish shell	130	N.A.	N.A.	8	70	7
⅙ deep dish made with vegetable shortening	140	N.A.	N.A.	9	80	0
⅙ graham cracker shell	110	N.A.	N.A.	6	50	7
tart shell (3″)	150	N.A.	N.A.	10	90	7

*Less than 2% U.S. RDA
†Frozen unless otherwise noted.

Sodium (mg)	Potassium (mg)	Protein (g)	Carbohy-drate (g)	Calcium (% U.S. RDA)	Iron (% U.S. RDA)	Vitamin A (% U.S. RDA)	Vitamin C (% U.S. RDA)
N.A.	N.A.	2	48	6	2	30	2
340	N.A.	3	43	2	10	*	2
60	N.A.	4	30	4	20	10	*
280	N.A.	3	35	*	6	4	25
380	N.A.	4	53	6	10	*	*
300	140	2	46	*	*	6	N.A.
190	N.A.	2	29	*	*	*	*
320	150	2	51	*	6	8	35
170	N.A.	2	41	*	4	2	20
260	N.A.	3	34	*	2	6	50
200	N.A.	3	51	2	2	*	*
290	N.A.	4	56	*	6	*	*
200	N.A.	4	31	*	6	4	*
140	15	1	10	*	2	*	*
110	25	1	11	*	N.A.	*	*
120	30	1	12	*	*	*	*
65	25	2	12	*	*	*	*
80	40	1	8	*	2	*	*
150	20	3	12	*	*	*	*

~ PIES & PASTRIES†	Calories	Saturated fat (g)	Polyunsat- urated fat (g)	Total fat (g)	Calories from fat	Choles- terol (mg)
Pillsbury All Ready, ready-to-use, ⅛ of two-crust pie	240	N.A.	N.A.	15	140	15
pie crust mix/sticks, 1/6 of two-crust pie	270	N.A.	N.A.	17	150	N.A.
Pop-Tarts, Kellogg, 1 pastry, all varieties	210	N.A.	N.A.	6	50	0
Puff pastry sheet, Pepperidge Farm, ¼ frozen sheet	260	N.A.	N.A.	17	150	N.A.
shell, 1 frozen	210	N.A.	N.A.	15	140	N.A.
Pumpkin pie						
Banquet family size, ⅙ of 20-oz pie	200	N.A.	N.A.	8	70	N.A.
canned mix (see Vegetables)						
Jell-O No Bake mix, ⅛ of pie	250	N.A.	N.A.	13	120	30
Mrs. Smith's pie in minutes, ⅛ of pie	190	2	1	6	50	35
Pet-Ritz pumpkin custard, ⅙ of 26-oz pie	250	N.A.	N.A.	9	80	N.A.
Sara Lee homestyle, ⅒ of 9″ pie	240	N.A.	N.A.	10	90	40
Raspberry pie, Sara Lee home- style, ⅒ of 9″ pie	280	N.A.	N.A.	13	120	0
Raspberry turnover, Pepper- idge Farm, 1 pastry	320	N.A.	N.A.	18	160	N.A.
Strawberry pie						
Banquet strawberry cream, ⅙ of 14-oz pie	170	N.A.	N.A.	9	80	N.A.
Hostess packaged snack pie, 1 pie	340	N.A.	N.A.	16	140	10
Pet-Ritz strawberry cream, ⅙ of 14-oz pie	170	N.A.	N.A.	9	80	N.A.
Sweet potato pie, Pet-Ritz, ⅙ of 20-oz pie	150	N.A.	N.A.	7	60	N.A.

*Less than 2% U.S. RDA
†Frozen unless otherwise noted.

Sodium (mg)	Potassium (mg)	Protein (g)	Carbohy-drate (g)	Calcium (% U.S. RDA)	Iron (% U.S. RDA)	Vitamin A (% U.S. RDA)	Vitamin C (% U.S. RDA)
210	30	2	24	*	*	*	*
420	80	4	25	*	6	*	*
210	60	2	36	*	10	10	*
290	N.A.	4	22	*	4	*	*
180	N.A.	2	17	*	2	*	*
350	N.A.	3	29	6	6	40	4
450	140	4	31	10	2	6	*
230	N.A.	3	30	4	10	*	*
N.A.	N.A.	4	39	2	6	*	15
250	N.A.	4	34	6	6	70	*
150	N.A.	2	39	*	6	*	4
270	N.A.	3	37	*	4	*	15
120	N.A.	2	22	4	6	*	10
400	N.A.	5	56	6	8	*	*
150	60	2	20	2	6	*	*
110	60	2	21	*	4	35	4

~ PIES & PASTRIES†/ PUDDINGS‡	Calories	Saturated fat (g)	Polyunsat- urated fat (g)	Total fat (g)	Calories from fat	Choles- terol (mg)
Vanilla pudding pie, Hostess snack pie, 1 pie	470	N.A.	N.A.	17	150	18
Chocolate mousse						
Duncan Hines Tiara Dessert, 1/12 dessert, chocolate, black forest, chocolate amaretto	270	N.A.	N.A.	15	140	N.A.
Jell-O No Bake mix, ½ cup	150	N.A.	N.A.	6	50	10
Pepperidge Farm American Collection, frozen, San Francisco chocolate mousse, 1 pkg	490	N.A.	N.A.	34	310	N.A.
Sara Lee Classics, frozen, 1/8 pkg	260	N.A.	N.A.	17	150	20
Lights, 1 pkg	170	N.A.	N.A.	8	70	10
Weight Watchers, frozen, ½ of pkg	170	<1	2	6	50	5
mix, ½ cup, all varieties	60	N.A.	N.A.	3	25	N.A.
Praline pecan mousse, Weight Watchers, frozen, ½ pkg	190	1	2	7	60	5
Pudding mix, regular Jell-O, ½ cup, all flavors	160	N.A.	N.A.	4	35	15
Americana, ½ cup, all flavors (egg custard con- tains 80 mg cholesterol)	160	N.A.	N.A.	4	35	15
microwave, ½ cup, all flavors	160	N.A.	N.A.	4	35	15
pudding and pie filling, 1/6 mix, banana cream, coconut cream	110	N.A.	N.A.	4	35	10
lemon	170	N.A.	N.A.	2	18	90
sugar-free, ½ cup prepared with 2% lowfat milk, chocolate, vanilla	90	N.A.	N.A.	3	25	10
Pudding mix, instant, Jell-O, ½ cup, all flavors	170	N.A.	N.A.	5	45	15

*Less than 2% U.S. RDA
†Frozen unless otherwise noted.
‡Packaged unless otherwise noted.

Sodium (mg)	Potassium (mg)	Protein (g)	Carbohy-drate (g)	Calcium (% U.S. RDA)	Iron (% U.S. RDA)	Vitamin A (% U.S. RDA)	Vitamin C (% U.S. RDA)
400	N.A.	4	75	10	10	*	*
250	N.A.	3	30	4	2	*	*
75	290	5	21	10	4	*	*
75	N.A.	4	41	8	4	*	*
100	N.A.	3	23	4	8	8	2
60	N.A.	4	20	15	6	6	*
190	210	6	24	6	6	*	8
40	N.A.	3	7	15	*	*	*
180	130	5	27	6	10	*	*
170	240	4	28	15	*	2	*
180	220	5	27	15	*	2	*
190	230	4	27	15	*	2	*
150	135	3	17	10	*	2	*
95	25	2	38	*	2	*	*
180	250	5	12	15	*	4	*
410	220	4	29	15	*	2	*

~ PUDDINGS†

	Calories	Saturated fat (g)	Polyunsaturated fat (g)	Total fat (g)	Calories from fat	Cholesterol (mg)
sugar-free, ½ cup prepared with 2% lowfat milk	90	N.A.	N.A.	3	25	10
Pudding mix, reduced calorie, D-Zerta, ½ cup, all varieties	70	0	0	0	0	0
Weight Watchers instant, ½ cup, all varieties	90	N.A.	N.A.	1	10	N.A.
Pudding, ready-to-eat						
Hershey's pudding pack, 4-oz cup, all varieties	180	N.A.	N.A.	5	45	N.A.
Hunt Snack Pack, 4.25 oz, all flavors	160	1	<1	6	50	1
Lite, 4 oz, chocolate, tapioca	100	<1	<1	2	18	1
Jell-O Pudding Snacks, 4 oz, all flavors	170	N.A.	N.A.	6	50	0
light, 4 oz, all flavors	100	N.A.	N.A.	2	18	5
Swiss Miss, ½ cup, all varieties	190	1	<1	6	50	2
light pudding, ½ cup, all flavors	100	<1	<1	1	10	<1
Raspberry mousse, Weight Watchers, frozen, ½ pkg	150	<1	2	6	50	5
mix, ½ cup	60	N.A.	N.A.	3	25	N.A.

*Less than 2% U.S. RDA
†Packaged unless otherwise noted.

Sodium (mg)	Potassium (mg)	Protein (g)	Carbohy-drate (g)	Calcium (% U.S. RDA)	Iron (% U.S. RDA)	Vitamin A (% U.S. RDA)	Vitamin C (% U.S. RDA)
380	230	4	12	15	*	4	*
65	250	4	12	15	*	4	2
460	N.A.	5	17	25	*	6	*
230	N.A.	3	29	10	*	2	*
140	100	2	26	6	*	2	*
115	150	3	19	8	*	4	*
135	220	3	28	10	*	2	*
125	170	3	21	8	*	4	*
160	180	3	29	10	4	*	*
115	160	3	20	8	*	2	*
150	140	5	21	4	2	2	2
75	N.A.	3	12	20	*	4	*

～ENTREES

～& SIDE DISHES

～ The first section lists frozen breakfast entrees. Regular entrees are frozen unless otherwise designated. Values for fiber and sugar content are not available. Most of these listings are from the manufacturer or from food labels and represent the most up-to-date information at this writing. Products are continually reformulated, however, and labels of products you use often should be checked occasionally.

~ BREAKFAST, FROZEN	Calories	Saturated fat (g)	Polyunsaturated fat (g)	Total fat (g)	Calories from fat	Cholesterol (mg)
Belgian waffle and sausage, Swanson Great Starts	280	N.A.	N.A.	19	170	N.A.
Egg, meat, and cheese on a muffin						
Swanson Great Starts, with beefsteak	380	N.A.	N.A.	22	200	N.A.
with Canadian bacon	300	N.A.	N.A.	16	140	N.A.
Weight Watchers, with Canadian bacon	230	1	1	8	70	170
Egg, meat, and cheese on a biscuit						
Swanson Great Starts, with Canadian bacon	420	N.A.	N.A.	22	200	N.A.
with sausage	470	N.A.	N.A.	29	260	N.A.
Eggs, scrambled						
Aunt Jemima Homestyle Breakfast, with sausage and hash browns	290	N.A.	N.A.	20	180	N.A.
Swanson Great Starts, with cheese and sweet roll	290	N.A.	N.A.	23	210	N.A.
with home fries	280	N.A.	N.A.	21	190	N.A.
with home fries and bacon	340	N.A.	N.A.	26	230	N.A.
with sausage and hash browns	420	N.A.	N.A.	34	310	N.A.
Egg and sausage substitutes (Scramblers, Breakfast Links), Morningstar Farms Country Breakfast, with hash browns	360	N.A.	N.A.	23	210	0
with pancakes	380	N.A.	N.A.	19	170	0
French toast						
Aunt Jemima, 2 slices, all varieties	230	N.A.	N.A.	7	60	N.A
French toast sticks with syrup	400	N.A.	N.A.	20	180	N.A.

*Less than 2% U.S. RDA

Sodium (mg)	Potassium (mg)	Protein (g)	Carbohy-drate (g)	Calcium (% U.S. RDA)	Iron (% U.S. RDA)	Vitamin A (% U.S. RDA)	Vitamin C (% U.S. RDA)
420	N.A.	7	21	4	6	*	2
770	N.A.	18	27	10	15	4	*
780	N.A.	14	25	10	10	2	*
610	210	13	26	15	6	2	*
1850	N.A.	16	37	25	25	*	2
1390	N.A.	17	34	15	10	6	*
810	300	12	14	8	8	6	6
380	N.A.	7	14	6	10	*	*
460	N.A.	7	15	4	8	2	2
680	N.A.	10	16	6	8	*	*
780	N.A.	12	16	6	10	*	2
660	160	16	22	2	25	15	4
900	170	18	33	4	15	8	4
350	135	8	34	8	15	4	*
640	115	7	48	8	10	2	*

~ BREAKFAST, FROZEN/ DINNER	Calories	Saturated fat (g)	Polyunsat- urated fat (g)	Total fat (g)	Calories from fat	Choles- terol (mg)
Morningstar Farms, with simulated sausage	380	N.A.	N.A.	15	140	0
Swanson Great Starts, plain, with sausage	460	N.A.	N.A.	26	230	N.A.
Weight Watchers, ½ of 6-oz pkg	160	<1	<1	4	35	5
with links, 4.5-oz pkg	270	3	2	11	100	15
Omelet, Swanson Great Starts, Spanish style	240	N.A.	N.A.	16	140	N.A.
with cheese sauce and ham	380	N.A.	N.A.	29	260	N.A.
Pancakes						
Aunt Jemima Homestyle Breakfast, with sausage	420	N.A.	N.A.	16	140	N.A.
Swanson Great Starts, with blueberries or strawberries	420	N.A.	N.A.	11	100	N.A.
with sausage	460	N.A.	N.A.	22	200	N.A.
Weight Watchers, butter- milk, ½ of 5-oz pkg	140	1	<1	3	25	10
with blueberry or strawberry topping	200	1	1	3	25	10
with links, 4-oz pkg	220	4	3	10	90	15
Beans and frankfurters						
Banquet dinner	520	N.A.	N.A.	25	230	35
Swanson 3-compartment dinner	440	N.A.	N.A.	20	180	N.A.
Beef and BBQ sauce						
Banquet Cookin' Bag, 4 oz	100	N.A.	N.A.	2	18	N.A.
Swanson 4-compartment dinner	460	N.A.	N.A.	15	140	N.A.
Beef Burgundy, Le Menu en- tree	330	N.A.	N.A.	23	210	N.A.
Beef champignon, Tyson Gourmet Selection Dinner	370	N.A.	N.A.	15	140	N.A.
Beef chop suey, Stouffer's en- tree, with rice	300	N.A.	N.A.	9	80	N.A.

*Less than 2% U.S. RDA

Sodium (mg)	Potassium (mg)	Protein (g)	Carbohy-drate (g)	Calcium (% U.S. RDA)	Iron (% U.S. RDA)	Vitamin A (% U.S. RDA)	Vitamin C (% U.S. RDA)
1220	270	24	37	10	25	8	*
650	N.A.	16	42	10	20	*	*
280	100	8	24	6	4	2	*
550	230	15	24	6	8	6	8
800	N.A.	8	15	8	10	10	20
1200	N.A.	18	12	25	10	10	2
1140	190	12	57	25	20	*	*
830	N.A.	8	73	8	15	*	8
900	N.A.	14	52	8	15	*	*
270	150	5	22	6	4	*	*
330	160	5	37	8	6	6	10
510	280	12	21	8	8	2	*
1230	790	17	57	10	25	90	50
900	N.A.	11	55	10	15	4	6
N.A.	N.A.	9	11	N.A.	N.A.	N.A.	N.A.
850	N.A.	29	51	6	25	35	6
660	N.A.	25	5	2	15	30	2
830	N.A.	27	31	N.A.	N.A.	N.A.	N.A.
1170	280	16	38	2	8	2	15

～ DINNER

	Calories	Saturated fat (g)	Polyunsaturated fat (g)	Total fat (g)	Calories from fat	Cholesterol (mg)
Beef chow mein, La Choy Bi-pack, ¾ cup beef, beef pepper	80	<1	<1	2	18	19
Beef, chopped, Banquet dinner	420	N.A.	N.A.	32	290	80
Beef, creamed chipped						
Banquet Cookin' Bag, 4 oz	100	N.A.	N.A.	4	35	N.A.
Stouffer's entree, ½ pkg	230	N.A.	N.A.	16	140	N.A.
Beef Dijon, Right Course, with pasta and vegetables	290	2	1	9	80	40
Beef dinner						
Banquet platter	460	N.A.	N.A.	34	310	75
Extra Helping	870	N.A.	N.A.	61	550	120
Swanson 4-compartment dinner	340	N.A.	N.A.	8	70	N.A.
Hungry Man dinner	450	N.A.	N.A.	12	110	N.A.
Beef, fiesta, Right Course, with corn pasta	270	2	2	7	60	30
Beef goulash, Heinz, ½ of 15-oz can	240	N.A.	N.A.	11	100	N.A.
Beef and gravy, Banquet Cookin' Bag						
sliced beef, gravy, 4 oz	100	N.A.	N.A.	5	45	N.A.
charbroiled patty, mushroom gravy, 5 oz	210	N.A.	N.A.	15	140	N.A.
Beef Mexicana, Budget Gourmet 3-dish dinner	560	N.A.	N.A.	23	210	50
Beef, Oriental						
Budget Gourmet Slim Selects	290	N.A.	N.A.	9	80	25
Lean Cuisine entree, with vegetables and rice	250	2	<1	7	60	45
Beef pie						
Banquet	510	N.A.	N.A.	33	300	25
microwave, single crust	440	N.A.	N.A.	29	260	35

*Less than 2% U.S. RDA

Sodium (mg)	Potassium (mg)	Protein (g)	Carbohy-drate (g)	Calcium (% U.S. RDA)	Iron (% U.S. RDA)	Vitamin A (% U.S. RDA)	Vitamin C (% U.S. RDA)
900	210	7	9	2	10	20	35
600	460	21	14	4	20	180	6
N.A.	N.A.	7	9	N.A.	N.A.	N.A.	N.A.
850	300	12	9	10	6	*	2
580	270	20	31	4	15	25	2
630	510	22	20	4	20	100	15
810	910	34	50	6	40	80	30
800	N.A.	27	41	4	25	6	8
1060	N.A.	37	49	4	25	10	10
590	430	18	33	6	15	15	10
920	N.A.	13	22	*	10	N.A.	N.A.
N.A.	N.A.	8	5	N.A.	N.A.	N.A.	N.A.
N.A.	N.A.	9	8	N.A.	N.A.	N.A.	N.A.
1290	N.A.	33	56	30	25	6	10
810	N.A.	17	36	6	10	15	15
900	250	18	28	2	8	15	*
870	190	12	39	4	15	10	2
730	220	14	30	4	15	15	4

∼ DINNER

	Calories	Saturated fat (g)	Polyunsaturated fat (g)	Total fat (g)	Calories from fat	Cholesterol (mg)
Stouffer's entree	500	N.A.	N.A.	32	290	N.A.
Swanson Pot Pie	380	N.A.	N.A.	20	180	N.A.
Hungry Man	700	N.A.	N.A.	36	320	N.A.
Worthington Foods vegetarian, 8 oz	360	N.A.	N.A.	16	140	0
Beef ragout, Right Course, with rice pilaf	300	2	1	8	70	50
Beef roast, Hormel Top Shelf	250	N.A.	N.A.	7	60	55
Beef short ribs						
Armour Classics dinner, boneless	380	N.A.	N.A.	16	140	90
Stouffer's entree, in gravy	350	N.A.	N.A.	20	180	N.A.
Tyson Gourmet Selection Dinner	470	N.A.	N.A.	24	220	N.A.
Beef stew						
Banquet family entree, ¼ of 28-oz pkg	140	N.A.	N.A.	5	45	N.A.
Heinz, ½ of 15-oz can	210	N.A.	N.A.	9	80	N.A.
Snoopy's Choice, Healthy Choice for Kids	140	1	<1	2	18	35
Worthington Foods, simulated beef, ½ of 19.5-oz can	220	1	6	10	90	0
Beef Stroganoff						
Armour Classics Lite dinner	250	N.A.	N.A.	6	50	55
Budget Gourmet Slim Selects	280	N.A.	N.A.	10	90	60
Le Menu dinner	450	N.A.	N.A.	25	230	N.A.
Stouffer's entree, with parsley noodles	390	N.A.	N.A.	20	180	N.A.
Weight Watchers entree	290	4	2	9	80	25
Worthington Foods, meatless mix (Natural Touch), ¼ of pouch	90	N.A.	N.A.	3	25	N.A.
Beef, Szechwan, Lean Cuisine entree, with noodles and vegetables	260	3	2	10	90	100

*Less than 2% U.S. RDA

Sodium (mg)	Potassium (mg)	Protein (g)	Carbohy-drate (g)	Calcium (% U.S. RDA)	Iron (% U.S. RDA)	Vitamin A (% U.S. RDA)	Vitamin C (% U.S. RDA)
1300	300	20	33	4	15	70	4
700	N.A.	11	37	2	15	25	2
1530	N.A.	27	66	2	30	50	8
1940	115	9	44	*	8	*	*
550	320	19	38	4	10	20	10
940	N.A.	27	20	4	20	35	15
790	770	24	34	6	25	15	30
900	400	30	12	4	15	40	6
950	N.A.	25	38	N.A.	N.A.	N.A.	N.A.
N.A.	N.A.	6	18	N.A.	N.A.	N.A.	N.A.
1250	N.A.	12	19	2	10	N.A.	N.A.
300	320	13	16	2	6	20	6
760	300	10	23	4	15	*	*
510	320	18	33	6	15	60	70
560	N.A.	18	29	6	15	4	15
1000	N.A.	25	30	10	20	10	2
1090	300	24	28	6	15	4	2
600	350	22	26	8	15	6	6
N.A.	N.A.	4	10	N.A.	N.A.	N.A.	N.A.
680	320	20	22	4	10	25	20

~ DINNER

	Calories	Saturated fat (g)	Polyunsat-urated fat (g)	Total fat (g)	Calories from fat	Choles-terol (mg)
Beef teriyaki, Stouffer's entree	290	N.A.	N.A.	8	70	N.A.
Beefsteak ranchero, Lean Cuisine entree	270	3	1	9	80	40
Burrito						
Old El Paso individual, all varieties	340	N.A.	N.A.	14	130	N.A.
Beef and Bean dinner	470	N.A.	N.A.	9	80	N.A.
Dinner Kit (with filling), 1 burrito	300	4	2	13	120	23
Weight Watchers entree, all varieties	310	4	3	13	120	65
Cabbage, stuffed, Lean Cuisine entree	220	2	0	10	90	55
Cannelloni						
Lean Cuisine entree, all varieties	260	5	1	10	90	40
Le Menu Light Style Dinner, chicken	270	N.A.	N.A.	5	45	N.A.
Cheese Beef Patty Sandwich, Kid Cuisine	400	N.A.	N.A.	19	170	40
Chefwich, microwave, Tetley, all varieties	370	N.A.	N.A.	13	120	27
Chicken, BBQ						
Stouffer's dinner	390	N.A.	N.A.	23	210	N.A.
Swanson 4-compartment dinner	460	N.A.	N.A.	13	120	N.A.
Tyson Looney Tunes Meals, Yosemite Sam	420	N.A.	N.A.	21	190	N.A.
Chicken and Beef Luau, Tyson Gourmet Selection Dinner	330	N.A.	N.A.	10	90	N.A.
Chicken Burgundy, Armour Classics Lite	210	N.A.	N.A.	2	18	45
Chicken cacciatore						
Budget Gourmet, 3-dish dinner	300	N.A.	N.A.	13	120	60

*Less than 2% U.S. RDA

Sodium (mg)	Potassium (mg)	Protein (g)	Carbohy-drate (g)	Calcium (% U.S. RDA)	Iron (% U.S. RDA)	Vitamin A (% U.S. RDA)	Vitamin C (% U.S. RDA)
1450	380	22	33	4	10	2	15
950	430	16	30	4	8	6	10
730	250	14	40	10	20	*	*
1180	480	23	72	15	35	4	*
430	220	11	36	4	10	*	2
790	430	16	35	8	15	8	6
930	530	14	19	6	10	15	10
930	370	19	23	25	6	20	6
590	N.A.	15	38	8	15	30	10
550	360	12	47	15	15	*	4
770	240	15	49	15	15	*	4
1250	650	22	24	15	10	8	15
940	N.A.	28	57	6	15	15	6
750	N.A.	28	30	N.A.	N.A.	N.A.	N.A.
1030	N.A.	18	42	N.A.	N.A.	N.A.	N.A.
780	510	23	25	4	15	40	40
810	N.A.	20	27	15	10	4	35

~ DINNER

	Calories	Saturated fat (g)	Polyunsat- urated fat (g)	Total fat (g)	Calories from fat	Choles- terol (mg)
Hunt's Minute Gourmet, ¼ pkg	280	N.A.	N.A.	6	50	N.A.
Le Menu Light Style dinner	270	3	1	8	70	85
Lean Cuisine entree, with vermicelli	250	1	2	7	60	45
Swanson homestyle entree	260	N.A.	N.A.	8	70	N.A.
Chicken, cashew, Stouffer's entree, with rice	380	N.A.	N.A.	16	140	N.A.
Chicken chow mein						
Armour Dining Light dinner, with rice	180	N.A.	N.A.	2	18	30
Healthy Choice entree	220	1	1	3	25	45
La Choy Bi-Pack, ¾ cup	80	<1	<1	3	25	18
dinner	300	2	8	17	150	16
Le Menu Light Style dinner	260	N.A.	N.A.	4	35	N.A.
Lean Cuisine entree, with rice	250	1	1	5	45	35
Stouffer's entree, no noodles	130	N.A.	N.A.	4	35	N.A.
Chicken chunks, Tyson Chick'n Chunks, 2.6 oz	220	N.A.	N.A.	15	140	35
breast chunks, 3 oz	240	N.A.	N.A.	17	150	30
Chicken chunks, Looney Tunes Meals, Bugs Bunny	370	N.A.	N.A.	20	180	N.A.
Chicken Cordon Bleu						
Le Menu dinner	470	N.A.	N.A.	20	180	N.A.
Weight Watchers entree	220	5	1	9	80	50
Chicken, creamed, Stouffer's entree	300	N.A.	N.A.	21	190	N.A.
Chicken in cream sauce, Lean Cuisine entree	260	3	2	10	90	80
Chicken croquettes						
Howard Johnson's, ½ of 12-oz pkg	400	N.A.	N.A.	19	170	63
Weaver, 2 croquettes	280	N.A.	N.A.	16	140	N.A.

*Less than 2% U.S. RDA

Sodium (mg)	Potassium (mg)	Protein (g)	Carbohy-drate (g)	Calcium (% U.S. RDA)	Iron (% U.S. RDA)	Vitamin A (% U.S. RDA)	Vitamin C (% U.S. RDA)
840	N.A.	35	20	20	15	6	15
640	N.A.	21	28	10	10	100	25
860	600	21	26	6	15	10	15
1030	N.A.	15	33	8	15	15	35
1140	530	31	29	2	10	2	2
650	180	10	31	2	6	*	8
440	290	18	31	2	8	8	6
970	225	7	8	2	4	10	25
1800	240	12	29	8	20	15	6
830	N.A.	18	37	6	8	10	8
980	300	14	36	4	4	2	15
1080	230	13	11	2	4	8	20
500	N.A.	10	11	N.A.	N.A.	N.A.	N.A.
430	N.A.	13	10	N.A.	N.A.	N.A.	N.A.
770	N.A.	17	31	N.A.	N.A.	N.A.	N.A.
870	N.A.	23	49	10	8	150	6
630	370	19	14	15	6	8	6
670	200	19	8	8	4	*	*
910	460	26	17	10	6	25	4
770	220	20	N.A.	*	N.A.	N.A.	N.A.
780	N.A.	14	22	N.A.	N.A.	N.A.	N.A.

	Calories	Saturated fat (g)	Polyunsat- urated fat (g)	Total fat (g)	Calories from fat	Choles- terol (mg)
½ cup gravy	25	N.A.	N.A.	2	18	N.A.
Chicken dinner						
Armour Classics, with wine and mushroom sauce	280	N.A.	N.A.	11	100	50
Stouffer's, baked breast	300	N.A.	N.A.	11	100	N.A.
with supreme sauce	360	N.A.	N.A.	12	110	N.A.
Swanson Hungry Man, boneless	700	N.A.	N.A.	28	250	N.A.
Chicken divan, Stouffer's en- tree	320	N.A.	N.A.	20	180	N.A.
Chicken Drumsnacker Platter, Banquet	430	N.A.	N.A.	19	170	N.A.
Chicken Duet, Swanson en- trees, all varieties	330	N.A.	N.A.	19	170	N.A.
Chicken and dumplings						
Banquet dinner	430	N.A.	N.A.	24	220	45
Swanson, 7½-oz canned	220	N.A.	N.A.	12	110	N.A.
Chicken, fiesta, Lean Cuisine entree	250	1	2	6	50	45
Chicken Florentine						
Le Menu dinner	340	N.A.	N.A.	10	90	N.A.
Stouffer's dinner	430	N.A.	N.A.	18	160	N.A.
Chicken français, Tyson Gour- met Selection dinner	280	N.A.	N.A.	14	130	N.A.
Chicken, French recipe, Budget Gourmet Slim Se- lects	260	N.A.	N.A.	10	90	60
Chicken, fried						
Banquet dinner	400	N.A.	N.A.	22	200	N.A.
Extra Helping dinner	570	N.A.	N.A.	28	250	N.A.
White Meat platter	430	N.A.	N.A.	22	200	105
Kid Cuisine dinner	420	N.A.	N.A.	22	200	N.A.
Stouffer's dinner	450	N.A.	N.A.	23	210	N.A.
Swanson homestyle entree	380	N.A.	N.A.	21	190	N.A.

*Less than 2% U.S. RDA

Sodium (mg)	Potassium (mg)	Protein (g)	Carbohy-drate (g)	Calcium (% U.S. RDA)	Iron (% U.S. RDA)	Vitamin A (% U.S. RDA)	Vitamin C (% U.S. RDA)
260	N.A.	1	4	N.A.	N.A.	N.A.	N.A.
900	550	22	24	8	6	40	40
830	520	30	20	2	6	15	10
990	600	33	29	10	6	80	60
1530	N.A.	48	65	8	30	10	10
780	490	24	11	20	4	6	30
690	600	20	49	4	15	6	25
590	N.A.	21	20	10	6	*	2
940	460	17	34	6	15	70	12
960	N.A.	11	19	2	4	10	*
880	450	21	29	2	6	15	20
990	N.A.	23	38	15	8	40	4
930	560	33	32	20	10	120	10
1130	N.A.	19	20	N.A.	N.A.	N.A.	N.A.
790	N.A.	21	21	6	6	60	4
1100	480	15	45	4	6	10	15
1470	580	20	70	6	6	15	15
N.A.	600	38	21	2	15	8	20
1050	N.A.	15	41	4	15	*	6
990	590	25	35	10	8	35	35
1030	N.A.	18	30	4	10	*	8

	Calories	Saturated fat (g)	Polyunsat-urated fat (g)	Total fat (g)	Calories from fat	Choles-terol (mg)
Swanson 3-compartment dinner	340	N.A.	N.A.	16	140	N.A.
4-compartment dinner, all varieties	550	N.A.	N.A.	25	230	N.A.
Hungry Man dinner, dark meat	860	N.A.	N.A.	45	410	N.A.
white meat dinner	870	N.A.	N.A.	46	410	N.A.
Weight Watchers, Southern fried entree	320	7	2	16	140	65
Chicken, glazed						
Armour Classics dinner	300	N.A.	N.A.	16	140	60
Healthy Choice entree	230	1	1	3	25	50
Hormel Top Shelf, breast	190	N.A.	N.A.	2	18	40
Le Menu Light Style dinner, breast	270	2	1	6	50	70
Lean Cuisine entree, with vegetable rice	270	1	4	8	70	55
Chicken au gratin, Budget Gourmet Slim Selects	260	N.A.	N.A.	11	100	70
Chicken, imperial, Weight Watchers entree	240	1	1	3	25	35
Chicken Italiano, Right Course	280	2	2	8	70	45
Chicken Kiev						
Le Menu entree	530	N.A.	N.A.	39	350	N.A.
Tyson Gourmet Selection dinner	520	N.A.	N.A.	33	300	N.A.
Weight Watchers entree	230	3	1	9	80	30
Chicken à la king						
Armour Classics Lite dinner	290	N.A.	N.A.	7	60	55
Dining Light	240	N.A.	N.A.	7	60	40
Banquet Cookin' Bag, 4 oz	110	N.A.	N.A.	5	45	N.A.
Le Menu dinner	330	N.A.	N.A.	14	130	N.A.
Stouffer's entree, with rice	290	N.A.	N.A.	9	80	N.A.
Swanson, 5¼-oz canned	180	N.A.	N.A.	12	110	N.A.

*Less than 2% U.S. RDA

Sodium (mg)	Potassium (mg)	Protein (g)	Carbohy-drate (g)	Calcium (% U.S. RDA)	Iron (% U.S. RDA)	Vitamin A (% U.S. RDA)	Vitamin C (% U.S. RDA)
850	N.A.	8	39	4	10	120	2
1160	N.A.	23	56	6	15	4	2
1660	N.A.	36	77	6	20	*	8
2150	N.A.	35	80	8	20	*	8
690	260	17	27	2	10	8	8
960	400	15	24	4	6	8	20
340	370	22	28	*	6	*	*
820	N.A.	21	21	4	6	70	6
760	N.A.	26	27	8	10	30	20
810	390	26	23	2	4	2	4
820	N.A.	20	21	20	10	70	20
640	490	21	32	4	6	8	8
560	520	24	29	10	10	4	25
780	N.A.	20	24	4	10	40	2
1200	N.A.	16	40	N.A.	N.A.	N.A.	N.A.
610	260	13	23	2	4	10	15
630	370	19	38	8	15	50	110
780	220	14	30	6	8	*	8
N.A.	N.A.	8	9	N.A.	N.A.	N.A.	N.A.
810	N.A.	22	28	6	8	10	10
890	260	19	34	8	4	2	6
690	N.A.	10	9	4	4	*	*

～ DINNER

	Calories	Saturated fat (g)	Polyunsaturated fat (g)	Total fat (g)	Calories from fat	Cholesterol (mg)
Weight Watchers entree	240	3	2	6	50	20
Chicken, mandarin						
Budget Gourmet Slim Selects	290	N.A.	N.A.	6	50	25
Healthy Choice entree, with rice and broccoli	260	<1	<1	2	18	50
Chicken marsala						
Armour Classics Lite dinner	250	N.A.	N.A.	7	60	80
Budget Gourmet	500	N.A.	N.A.	5	45	65
Lean Cuisine entree, with vegetables	190	1	1	5	45	80
Tyson Gourmet Selection dinner	300	N.A.	N.A.	13	120	N.A.
Chicken mesquite						
Armour Classics dinner	370	N.A.	N.A.	16	140	55
Healthy Choice dinner	310	<1	<1	2	18	45
Tyson Gourmet Selection dinner	320	N.A.	N.A.	10	90	N.A.
Chicken Mexicana, Budget Gourmet 3-dish dinner	510	N.A.	N.A.	15	140	40
Chicken Nibbles, Swanson homestyle entree	340	N.A.	N.A.	24	220	N.A.
Chicken and noodles						
Armour Classics dinner	230	N.A.	N.A.	7	60	50
Dining Light	240	N.A.	N.A.	7	60	50
Budget Gourmet, with broccoli	450	N.A.	N.A.	26	230	130
Stouffer's entree, escalloped	420	N.A.	N.A.	25	230	N.A.
homestyle entree	310	N.A.	N.A.	15	140	N.A.
Weight Watchers homestyle entree	240	2	1	7	60	30
Chicken nuggets						
Banquet Hot Bites, ¼ of 10½-oz pkg, all varieties	230	N.A.	N.A.	16	140	N.A.

*Less than 2% U.S. RDA

Sodium (mg)	Potassium (mg)	Protein (g)	Carbohy-drate (g)	Calcium (% U.S. RDA)	Iron (% U.S. RDA)	Vitamin A (% U.S. RDA)	Vitamin C (% U.S. RDA)
490	260	17	28	15	4	8	15
690	N.A.	19	40	4	4	35	4
400	400	23	39	2	10	25	15
930	440	20	27	6	15	8	30
660	N.A.	15	37	4	15	20	6
400	850	25	11	2	6	25	15
900	N.A.	19	26	N.A.	N.A.	N.A.	N.A.
660	810	15	42	4	15	10	25
270	630	21	52	4	10	15	170
700	N.A.	23	35	N.A.	N.A.	N.A.	N.A.
1210	N.A.	23	70	25	60	6	20
480	N.A.	10	21	2	6	*	10
660	540	19	23	8	15	90	100
570	300	17	28	10	10	25	*
1110	N.A.	23	31	25	10	8	4
1230	250	21	27	10	8	2	*
1090	430	23	21	15	6	30	2
450	300	19	25	10	10	8	*
510	135	11	11	*	N.A.	*	4

	Calories	Saturated fat (g)	Polyunsaturated fat (g)	Total fat (g)	Calories from fat	Cholesterol (mg)
microwave, with sauce, 4.5 oz, all varieties	370	N.A.	N.A.	22	200	N.A.
Swanson Chicken Duet Gourmet Nuggets, 2.7 oz, ham & cheese	190	N.A.	N.A.	12	110	N.A.
Chicken nugget dinner						
Banquet Platter	430	N.A.	N.A.	21	190	N.A.
Extra Helping, with BBQ sauce	640	N.A.	N.A.	36	320	N.A.
Kid Cuisine	400	N.A.	N.A.	19	170	60
Swanson 4-compartment dinner	460	N.A.	N.A.	25	230	N.A.
Weight Watchers entree	270	4	2	12	110	50
Chicken à l'orange						
Healthy Choice entree	260	<1	<1	2	18	45
Lean Cuisine entree, with almond rice	260	1	1	5	45	55
Tyson Gourmet Selection dinner	300	N.A.	N.A.	8	70	N.A.
Chicken Oriental						
Armour Classics Lite dinner	180	N.A.	N.A.	1	10	35
Healthy Choice dinner	230	<1	<1	1	10	35
Le Menu entree	330	N.A.	N.A.	9	80	N.A.
Lean Cuisine entree	230	1	2	6	50	100
Tyson Gourmet Selection dinner	270	N.A.	N.A.	7	60	N.A.
Chicken parmigiana						
Armour Classics dinner	370	N.A.	N.A.	19	170	75
Budget Gourmet Light & Healthy dinner, breast	260	3	2	8	70	50
Healthy Choice dinner	280	2	<1	3	25	60
Le Menu dinner	400	N.A.	N.A.	20	180	N.A.
Lean Cuisine entree	260	2	2	8	70	80
Stouffer's dinner	360	N.A.	N.A.	15	140	N.A.

*Less than 2% U.S. RDA

Sodium (mg)	Potassium (mg)	Protein (g)	Carbohy-drate (g)	Calcium (% U.S. RDA)	Iron (% U.S. RDA)	Vitamin A (% U.S. RDA)	Vitamin C (% U.S. RDA)
840	280	20	22	*	6	*	6
370	N.A.	10	11	10	4	*	*
630	570	17	46	2	15	4	20
1390	770	29	56	4	20	8	25
610	400	11	46	2	15	*	6
710	N.A.	19	40	2	10	2	2
540	520	15	24	2	15	6	8
90	440	22	39	2	4	15	45
430	420	24	30	2	4	6	10
670	N.A.	21	36	N.A.	N.A.	N.A.	N.A.
660	510	18	24	4	6	10	80
460	450	19	36	4	10	6	50
820	N.A.	16	46	2	4	20	25
790	400	22	23	4	10	4	25
1140	N.A.	20	32	N.A.	N.A.	N.A.	N.A.
1060	540	22	27	15	20	20	15
420	440	22	29	15	8	100	45
310	620	23	38	10	15	90	60
900	N.A.	26	29	15	15	10	20
870	700	27	19	15	8	10	10
1150	750	31	25	25	10	15	10

	Calories	Saturated fat (g)	Polyunsaturated fat (g)	Total fat (g)	Calories from fat	Cholesterol (mg)
Tyson Gourmet Selection dinner	380	N.A.	N.A.	17	150	N.A.
Chicken and pasta, Healthy Choice dinner	310	2	<1	4	35	60
Chicken patty						
Banquet Platter	380	N.A.	N.A.	21	190	N.A.
Weight Watchers, Southern fried entree	340	4	3	16	140	50
Chicken piccata, Tyson Gourmet Selection dinner	240	N.A.	N.A.	10	90	N.A.
Chicken pie						
Banquet	550	N.A.	N.A.	36	320	35
microwave, single crust	430	N.A.	N.A.	28	250	40
Stouffer's entree	530	N.A.	N.A.	33	300	N.A.
Swanson homestyle entree	380	N.A.	N.A.	19	170	N.A.
Swanson Pot Pie	370	N.A.	N.A.	22	200	N.A.
Hungry Man	740	N.A.	N.A.	41	370	N.A.
Worthington Foods, simulated chicken, 8 oz	380	3	13	20	180	0
Chicken pieces						
Banquet, fried, ⅕ of 32-oz pkg	330	N.A.	N.A.	19	170	N.A.
breast portion, ½ of 11½-oz pkg	220	N.A.	N.A.	11	100	N.A.
thighs and drumsticks, ½ of 12½ oz pkg	250	N.A.	N.A.	14	130	N.A.
Weaver, Dutch Frye, crispy, 3.6 oz, assorted pieces	290	N.A.	N.A.	18	160	N.A.
Weaver, batter-dipped, breast, 4.4 oz	310	N.A.	N.A.	20	180	N.A.
drums and thighs, 3 oz	210	N.A.	N.A.	14	130	N.A.
wings, 3.6 oz	280	N.A.	N.A.	20	180	N.A.
Weaver, skinless breast, crispy, 2.9 oz	170	N.A.	N.A.	9	80	N.A.
Chicken, roasted						

*Less than 2% U.S. RDA

Sodium (mg)	Potassium (mg)	Protein (g)	Carbohy-drate (g)	Calcium (% U.S. RDA)	Iron (% U.S. RDA)	Vitamin A (% U.S. RDA)	Vitamin C (% U.S. RDA)
1100	N.A.	19	37	N.A.	N.A.	N.A.	N.A.
510	440	23	45	15	10	70	120
760	470	15	34	4	6	8	10
800	310	18	31	2	10	8	10
680	N.A.	19	19	N.A.	N.A.	N.A.	N.A.
860	190	15	39	4	15	6	*
740	230	15	30	4	6	15	4
1260	290	22	35	10	10	50	2
860	N.A.	13	40	4	8	30	4
810	N.A.	10	35	2	8	35	2
1630	N.A.	27	65	6	20	80	*
1200	105	7	43	2	8	*	*
1210	N.A.	18	29	2	6	2	*
710	N.A.	16	13	2	6	*	*
790	N.A.	14	14	*	6	*	*
550	N.A.	16	16	N.A.	N.A.	N.A.	N.A.
220	N.A.	20	13	N.A.	N.A.	N.A.	N.A.
220	N.A.	11	11	N.A.	N.A.	N.A.	N.A.
210	N.A.	13	13	N.A.	N.A.	N.A.	N.A.
320	N.A.	14	9	N.A.	N.A.	N.A.	N.A.

~ DINNER

	Calories	Saturated fat (g)	Polyunsaturated fat (g)	Total fat (g)	Calories from fat	Cholesterol (mg)
Budget Gourmet 3-dish dinner	280	N.A.	N.A.	7	60	40
Healthy Choice dinner	260	1	1	3	25	50
Le Menu Light Style dinner	220	3	1	6	50	55
Chicken, salsa, Healthy Choice dinner	240	1	<1	2	18	45
Chicken sandwich, Tyson Looney Tunes Meals, Road Runner	320	N.A.	N.A.	11	100	N.A.
Chicken, sesame, Right Course	320	2	4	9	80	50
Chicken stew						
Heinz, ½ of 15-oz can, with dumplings	210	N.A.	N.A.	9	80	N.A.
Swanson, ½ of 15¼-oz can	170	N.A.	N.A.	7	60	N.A.
Chicken, sweet and sour						
Armour Classics Lite dinner	240	N.A.	N.A.	2	18	35
Budget Gourmet, with rice	350	N.A.	N.A.	7	60	40
Healthy Choice dinner	280	<1	<1	2	18	50
La Choy Bi-Pack, ¾ cup	120	<1	<1	2	18	13
La Choy entree	240	<1	<1	2	18	19
dinner	450	N.A.	N.A.	22	200	N.A.
Swanson 4-compartment dinner	380	N.A.	N.A.	11	100	N.A.
Tyson Gourmet Selection dinner	420	N.A.	N.A.	15	140	N.A.
Chicken tenderloins, Right Course, in BBQ sauce	270	1	2	6	50	40
in peanut sauce	330	2	3	10	90	50
Chicken tenders						
Tyson, Southern fried breast, 3 oz	220	N.A.	N.A.	11	100	25
microwave tenders, 3.5 oz	230	N.A.	N.A.	11	100	N.A.
Weaver, 3 oz, all varieties	180	N.A.	N.A.	9	80	N.A.

*Less than 2% U.S. RDA

Sodium (mg)	Potassium (mg)	Protein (g)	Carbohy-drate (g)	Calcium (% U.S. RDA)	Iron (% U.S. RDA)	Vitamin A (% U.S. RDA)	Vitamin C (% U.S. RDA)
1110	N.A.	19	34	10	15	*	15
300	500	20	38	2	8	15	210
610	N.A.	21	21	4	8	10	10
400	540	20	36	8	6	20	110
610	N.A.	9	46	N.A.	N.A.	N.A.	N.A.
590	400	25	34	4	10	10	20
850	N.A.	9	22	4	6	N.A.	N.A.
960	N.A.	9	16	2	4	110	10
820	490	18	39	4	6	20	45
640	N.A.	18	53	6	4	8	4
260	470	22	44	4	8	6	140
440	400	7	18	2	10	40	25
1420	240	8	47	2	10	35	6
1170	N.A.	20	42	8	10	35	10
520	N.A.	20	50	8	6	15	10
850	N.A.	22	50	N.A.	N.A.	N.A.	N.A.
590	590	20	35	6	8	35	45
570	470	27	32	8	10	6	10
630	N.A.	14	15	N.A.	N.A.	N.A.	N.A.
600	N.A.	16	19	N.A.	N.A.	N.A.	N.A.
500	N.A.	12	12	N.A.	N.A.	N.A.	N.A.

	Calories	Saturated fat (g)	Polyunsat-urated fat (g)	Total fat (g)	Calories from fat	Choles-terol (mg)
Weight Watchers entree, Sweet 'n Sour	240	<1	<1	1	10	40
Chicken teriyaki						
Budget Gourmet 3-dish dinner	360	N.A.	N.A.	12	110	55
Light & Healthy dinner, breast	310	1	4	9	80	30
La Choy Bi-Pack, ¾ cup	90	<1	<1	2	18	20
Chicken and vegetables						
Banquet Cookin' Bag, 4 oz	100	N.A.	N.A.	2	18	N.A.
Healthy Choice entree	210	<1	<1	1	10	35
Lean Cuisine entree, with vermicelli	270	2	2	8	70	45
Chili						
canned						
Heinz, 1 cup	350	N.A.	N.A.	21	190	N.A.
with beans, hot, 1 cup	330	N.A.	N.A.	16	140	N.A.
Old El Paso, 1 cup	160	N.A.	N.A.	7	60	47
with beans, 1 cup	220	N.A.	N.A.	10	90	32
Van Camp's, 1 cup	410	N.A.	N.A.	34	310	N.A.
with beans, 1 cup	350	N.A.	N.A.	23	210	N.A.
Worthington Foods, meatless, ⅔ cup	190	1	6	10	90	0
spicy (Natural Touch), ⅔ cup	230	1	5	12	110	0
frozen						
Right Course, vegetarian, 1 pkg	280	1	2	7	60	0
Stouffer's entree	260	N.A.	N.A.	10	90	N.A.
Swanson homestyle entree	270	N.A.	N.A.	10	90	N.A.
packaged Fantastic Foods, vegetarian, ½ cup	100	N.A.	N.A.	<1	N.A.	N.A.
Chili dog, Hormel, with cheese	340	N.A.	N.A.	20	180	80

*Less than 2% U.S. RDA

Sodium (mg)	Potassium (mg)	Protein (g)	Carbohydrate (g)	Calcium (% U.S. RDA)	Iron (% U.S. RDA)	Vitamin A (% U.S. RDA)	Vitamin C (% U.S. RDA)
600	350	16	43	2	10	4	4
610	N.A.	20	44	8	8	30	20
440	390	19	41	4	4	25	60
850	230	8	8	2	6	20	20
N.A.	N.A.	6	14	N.A.	N.A.	N.A.	N.A.
490	390	20	31	4	15	15	15
980	400	20	29	10	8	20	20
1000	N.A.	15	27	6	20	N.A.	N.A.
1140	N.A.	15	30	10	15	N.A.	N.A.
510	550	19	8	4	15	40	N.A.
480	560	15	17	4	20	55	N.A.
1500	370	15	12	4	25	100	N.A.
1220	540	15	21	6	30	70	N.A.
550	180	10	15	*	6	*	*
890	470	12	19	8	15	*	*
590	600	9	45	8	10	20	25
1270	700	19	24	8	20	20	25
740	N.A.	20	26	6	20	25	6
180	N.A.	8	19	N.A.	N.A.	N.A.	N.A.
540	N.A.	14	25	10	10	10	10

～ DINNER

	Calories	Saturated fat (g)	Polyunsaturated fat (g)	Total fat (g)	Calories from fat	Cholesterol (mg)
Clams, light batter fried, Mrs. Paul's, 2½ oz	240	N.A.	N.A.	13	120	N.A.
Crab, deviled, Mrs. Paul's, 1 cake	170	N.A.	N.A.	7	60	N.A.
miniature, 3½ oz	250	N.A.	N.A.	12	110	N.A.
Egg foo young, La Choy Dinner Classics, 2 patties plus 3 oz sauce	160	2	4	7	60	275
Egg rolls						
La Choy, 3 oz, all varieties	150	<1	2	5	45	6
Van de Kamp's, Cantonese, 5¼ oz	280	N.A.	N.A.	5	45	N.A.
Worthington Foods, vegetarian, 3 oz	160	1	3	6	50	0
Eggplant parmigiana, Mrs. Paul's, frozen, ½ of 10-oz pkg	240	4	0	15	140	16
Enchanadas, Lean Cuisine entree, all varieties	280	2	2	10	90	63
Enchiladas						
Banquet						
beef dinner	500	N.A.	N.A.	15	140	N.A.
cheese dinner	550	N.A.	N.A.	19	170	N.A.
Family Entree, beef and chili gravy, ¼ of 28-oz pkg	270	N.A.	N.A.	13	120	N.A.
Budget Gourmet Slim Selects, chicken suiza	270	N.A.	N.A.	9	80	50
sirloin ranchero	290	N.A.	N.A.	15	140	35
Healthy Choice, chicken dinner	330	3	2	6	50	25
Old El Paso						
beef dinner	390	N.A.	N.A.	8	70	N.A.
entree, 1 enchilada	210	N.A.	N.A.	13	120	10
cheese dinner	590	N.A.	N.A.	31	280	N.A.

*Less than 2% U.S. RDA

Sodium (mg)	Potassium (mg)	Protein (g)	Carbohy-drate (g)	Calcium (% U.S. RDA)	Iron (% U.S. RDA)	Vitamin A (% U.S. RDA)	Vitamin C (% U.S. RDA)
380	N.A.	8	22	2	6	*	*
390	N.A.	8	19	10	6	*	*
480	N.A.	8	29	8	8	*	*
1250	270	8	19	6	10	25	*
330	200	6	21	4	8	6	20
550	N.A.	10	40	N.A.	N.A.	N.A.	N.A.
530	95	6	20	2	4	*	*
600	N.A.	6	18	10	6	*	100
870	440	16	32	15	15	25	10
1810	410	19	72	10	25	8	10
2170	420	22	71	30	20	15	10
N.A.	N.A.	10	28	N.A.	N.A.	N.A.	N.A.
1080	N.A.	17	30	20	30	15	2
770	N.A.	19	20	20	35	30	2
420	430	13	56	15	6	20	60
1200	600	24	56	15	25	2	*
720	330	8	16	10	8	*	15
1200	350	24	51	80	10	25	*

	Calories	Saturated fat (g)	Polyunsat-urated fat (g)	Total fat (g)	Calories from fat	Choles-terol (mg)
entree, 1 enchilada	250	N.A.	N.A.	12	110	N.A.
chicken dinner	460	N.A.	N.A.	18	160	N.A.
entree, 1 enchilada	220	N.A.	N.A.	12	110	N.A.
Dinner Kit (with filling), 1 enchilada	150	3	1	8	70	21
Stouffer's entree, cheese	590	N.A.	N.A.	40	360	N.A.
chicken entree	490	N.A.	N.A.	29	260	N.A.
Swanson 4-compartment dinner, beef	480	N.A.	N.A.	22	200	N.A.
Tyson Looney Tunes, beef, Speedy Gonzales	400	N.A.	N.A.	16	140	N.A.
Weight Watchers entree, beef ranchero	230	3	2	10	90	40
cheese ranchero	360	5	2	18	160	60
chicken suiza	280	2	2	11	100	30
Fajitas						
Healthy Choice Mexican entree, beef	210	2	1	4	35	35
chicken	200	1	1	3	25	35
Weight Watchers entree, beef	250	2	1	7	60	20
chicken	230	2	1	5	45	30
Fettuccine						
Armour Classics, chicken	260	N.A.	N.A.	9	80	50
Dining Light, with alfredo sauce and broccoli	290	N.A.	N.A.	12	110	35
Budget Gourmet, chicken	400	N.A.	N.A.	21	190	100
Light & Healthy dinner, chicken breast	240	3	1	7	60	55
Slim Selects, with meat sauce	290	N.A.	N.A.	10	90	25
Green Giant, primavera, microwave Garden Gourmet, 9.5-oz pkg	230	3	3	8	70	25

*Less than 2% U.S. RDA

Sodium (mg)	Potassium (mg)	Protein (g)	Carbohy-drate (g)	Calcium (% U.S. RDA)	Iron (% U.S. RDA)	Vitamin A (% U.S. RDA)	Vitamin C (% U.S. RDA)
830	340	10	24	25	8	*	*
770	520	21	54	10	20	4	15
740	340	8	20	15	8	*	2
330	180	7	11	4	6	2	4
880	440	23	34	60	8	15	10
910	490	22	34	30	6	6	4
1300	N.A.	16	54	15	15	30	6
830	N.A.	12	52	N.A.	N.A.	N.A.	N.A.
720	480	20	17	25	10	30	20
900	400	18	30	50	8	35	30
600	340	19	28	30	6	4	4
250	290	19	26	10	15	10	10
310	360	17	25	8	15	15	15
630	350	15	32	10	10	2	4
590	300	17	30	4	6	4	4
660	400	17	28	15	15	35	100
1020	250	12	33	20	15	6	35
740	N.A.	23	29	20	10	35	4
430	490	23	28	20	10	60	40
980	N.A.	16	34	10	15	100	4
610	250	13	26	15	10	15	20

～ DINNER

	Calories	Saturated fat (g)	Polyunsaturated fat (g)	Total fat (g)	Calories from fat	Cholesterol (mg)
Healthy Choice entree, alfredo	240	2	2	7	60	45
chicken	240	2	2	4	35	45
Stouffer's side dish, alfredo, ½ of 10-oz pkg	270	N.A.	N.A.	19	170	N.A.
Weight Watchers entree, alfredo	210	3	1	8	70	35
chicken	280	3	2	9	80	40
Fish 'n' Chips, Swanson 4-compartment dinner	500	N.A.	N.A.	20	180	N.A.
'n' Fries, homestyle entree	350	N.A.	N.A.	17	150	N.A.
Fish Dijon, Mrs. Paul's Light entree	200	2	0	5	45	N.A.
Fish divan, Lean Cuisine entree	260	2	1	7	60	85
Fish Florentine						
Lean Cuisine entree	230	2	2	8	70	100
Mrs. Paul's Light entree	220	4	0	8	70	N.A.
Fish au gratin						
Mrs. Paul's Light entree	270	N.A.	N.A.	9	80	N.A.
Weight Watchers entree	200	1	1	6	50	60
Fish jardiniere, Lean Cuisine entree	290	4	<1	10	90	110
Fish Mornay, Mrs. Paul's Light entree	230	4	0	10	90	N.A.
Fish nuggets						
Kid Cuisine	320	N.A.	N.A.	15	140	45
Swanson 4-compartment dinner	410	N.A.	N.A.	19	170	N.A.
Fish, oven-fried, Weight Watchers entree	240	<1	2	7	60	15
Fish and pasta Florentine, Mrs. Paul's Light entree	230	N.A.	N.A.	8	70	N.A.
Fish platter, Banquet	450	N.A.	N.A.	22	200	95
Fish portions, Mrs. Paul's						

*Less than 2% U.S. RDA

Sodium (mg)	Potassium (mg)	Protein (g)	Carbohydrate (g)	Calcium (% U.S. RDA)	Iron (% U.S. RDA)	Vitamin A (% U.S. RDA)	Vitamin C (% U.S. RDA)
370	70	10	36	10	10	*	*
370	190	22	29	8	10	*	*
560	100	8	17	15	2	2	*
600	570	17	18	30	6	8	6
590	240	22	25	20	10	4	*
930	N.A.	19	60	6	15	6	4
690	N.A.	15	35	2	10	*	2
650	N.A.	21	17	20	4	*	6
750	900	31	17	20	6	6	50
700	580	26	13	15	6	10	*
820	N.A.	25	10	40	6	2	8
430	N.A.	35	14	25	30	4	*
700	520	25	11	15	4	6	15
840	900	31	18	15	2	20	*
670	N.A.	24	12	30	4	2	35
750	290	13	33	8	15	2	4
930	N.A.	17	43	4	10	30	*
380	340	20	23	2	4	10	8
870	N.A.	18	21	25	6	4	6
N.A.	980	31	33	8	15	8	25

～ DINNER

	Calories	Saturated fat (g)	Polyunsaturated fat (g)	Total fat (g)	Calories from fat	Cholesterol (mg)
batter-dipped fillets, 2	430	4	7	28	250	50
buttered fillets, 2	160	5	1	8	70	105
cakes, 2	250	N.A.	N.A.	11	100	N.A.
crispy crunchy fillets, 2	220	2	2	9	80	22
crispy crunchy sticks, 4	190	1	2	8	70	25
crunchy batter fillets, 2	280	3	3	14	130	22
light fillets, ½ of 9-oz pkg	250	N.A.	N.A.	9	80	N.A.
Fish sticks, Tyson Looney Tunes Meals, Sylvester	300	N.A.	N.A.	15	140	N.A.
Green Peppers, stuffed, Stouffer's entree, ½ of 15½-oz pkg	200	N.A.	N.A.	9	80	N.A.
Ham and asparagus bake, Stouffer's entree	510	N.A.	N.A.	35	320	N.A.
Ham and asparagus au gratin, Budget Gourmet Slim Selects	280	N.A.	N.A.	10	90	40
Ham platter, Banquet	400	N.A.	N.A.	17	150	50
Ham, scalloped potatoes and, Swanson homestyle entree	340	N.A.	N.A.	16	140	N.A.
Ham steak						
Armour Classics dinner	270	N.A.	N.A.	7	60	50
Le Menu dinner	300	N.A.	N.A.	10	90	N.A.
Stouffer's dinner	380	N.A.	N.A.	15	140	N.A.
Hamburger Helper, General Mills, ⅕ pkg prepared (*except* chili with beans = ¼ pkg; Pizzabake, Sloppy Joe, and Tacobake, *all* = ⅙ pkg)	340	N.A.	N.A.	17	150	N.A.
Hash, canned						
corned beef, with potatoes, 1 cup	410	11	N.A.	26	230	N.A.
roast beef, with potatoes, 1 cup, no added salt	290	N.A.	N.A.	10	90	N.A.
Lasagna						

*Less than 2% U.S. RDA

Sodium (mg)	Potassium (mg)	Protein (g)	Carbohy-drate (g)	Calcium (% U.S. RDA)	Iron (% U.S. RDA)	Vitamin A (% U.S. RDA)	Vitamin C (% U.S. RDA)
800	N.A.	17	27	4	2	*	*
230	N.A.	21	1	*	*	4	*
840	N.A.	11	27	6	8	*	*
380	N.A.	13	23	4	4	*	*
560	N.A.	9	18	4	4	*	*
730	N.A.	12	26	2	2	*	*
470	N.A.	17	23	4	4	*	*
670	N.A.	12	29	N.A.	N.A.	N.A.	N.A.
940	400	11	19	4	8	6	10
900	360	18	31	20	8	6	60
1130	N.A.	14	33	10	6	2	8
1180	490	20	43	4	15	140	20
990	N.A.	19	31	30	6	*	15
1320	640	15	36	15	15	4	10
1490	N.A.	18	33	6	10	160	40
1960	520	25	35	20	10	20	35
1040	440	23	30	4	15	6	*
1230	450	20	24	4	25	N.A.	N.A.
40	N.A.	22	29	4	15	*	35

	Calories	Saturated fat (g)	Polyunsaturated fat (g)	Total fat (g)	Calories from fat	Cholesterol (mg)
Banquet Family Entree, with meat sauce, ¼ of 28-oz pkg	270	N.A.	N.A.	10	90	N.A.
Budget Gourmet, Italian sausage	420	N.A.	N.A.	20	180	80
Slim Selects, with meat sauce	290	N.A.	N.A.	10	90	25
three-cheese	400	N.A.	N.A.	17	150	65
Healthy Choice entree, with meat sauce	250	2	1	4	35	20
zucchini	240	2	<1	3	25	15
Snoopy's Choice	280	3	2	7	60	25
Hormel Top Shelf, shelf-stable	360	N.A.	N.A.	16	140	70
Lean Cuisine entree, with meat and sauce	270	3	0	8	70	60
tuna with spinach noodles and vegetables	270	2	2	10	90	35
zucchini	260	2	0	7	60	25
Stouffer's entree	360	N.A.	N.A.	13	120	N.A.
fiesta	430	N.A.	N.A.	22	200	N.A.
vegetable	420	N.A.	N.A.	24	220	N.A.
Swanson homestyle entree, with meat sauce	400	N.A.	N.A.	16	140	N.A.
Weight Watchers entree, garden	290	2	2	7	60	20
Italian cheese	350	4	4	12	110	30
with meat sauce	320	4	2	10	90	45
Linguine						
Budget Gourmet Slim Selects, with scallops and clams	280	N.A.	N.A.	11	100	60
entree, with shrimp	330	N.A.	N.A.	15	140	75
Healthy Choice entree, with shrimp	230	1	1	2	18	55

*Less than 2% U.S. RDA

Sodium (mg)	Potassium (mg)	Protein (g)	Carbohy-drate (g)	Calcium (% U.S. RDA)	Iron (% U.S. RDA)	Vitamin A (% U.S. RDA)	Vitamin C (% U.S. RDA)
N.A.	N.A.	15	30	N.A.	N.A.	N.A.	N.A.
950	N.A.	20	38	40	15	100	*
890	N.A.	18	32	30	15	100	4
760	N.A.	22	38	50	15	100	4
420	500	16	38	10	15	15	50
390	830	16	37	25	15	35	10
490	840	15	39	8	20	35	10
1350	N.A.	24	30	30	10	20	4
970	550	25	24	20	10	8	10
890	440	17	29	25	8	40	6
950	600	20	28	30	8	30	10
1020	550	28	33	25	10	15	10
960	520	24	35	25	10	10	10
970	380	23	29	60	6	50	2
870	N.A.	25	39	45	15	10	8
670	600	19	35	30	15	25	20
690	770	29	33	70	10	35	30
630	760	26	32	40	15	35	35
630	N.A.	16	28	10	25	8	4
1250	N.A.	15	33	10	20	100	4
390	280	12	40	8	20	8	10

~ DINNER

	Calories	Saturated fat (g)	Polyunsaturated fat (g)	Total fat (g)	Calories from fat	Cholesterol (mg)
Lean Cuisine entree, with clam sauce	270	1	2	7	60	30
Lobster Newburg, Stouffer's entree	380	N.A.	N.A.	32	290	N.A.
London broil, Weight Watchers entree, mushroom sauce	140	1	1	3	25	40
Macaroni and beef						
Franco-American Hearty Pasta with Beef, ½ of 15-oz can	200	N.A.	N.A.	5	45	N.A.
Snoopy's Choice, Healthy Choice for Kids entree	250	2	1	5	45	15
Heinz, Mac 'n' Beef in Tomato Sauce, ½ of 14½-oz can	200	N.A.	N.A.	8	70	N.A.
Stouffer's entree, ½ of 11½-oz pkg	170	N.A.	N.A.	7	60	N.A.
Swanson 3-compartment dinner	370	N.A.	N.A.	15	140	N.A.
Macaroni and cheese						
Banquet 8-oz casserole	350	N.A.	N.A.	17	150	N.A.
dinner	420	N.A.	N.A.	20	180	30
Family Entree, ¼ of 32-oz pkg	290	N.A.	N.A.	13	120	N.A.
Budget Gourmet side dish	210	N.A.	N.A.	8	70	25
Franco American, 1 cup canned	170	N.A.	N.A.	5	45	N.A.
Heinz, 1 cup canned	190	N.A.	N.A.	8	70	N.A.
Howard Johnson's, ½ of 10-oz pkg	180	N.A.	N.A.	8	70	15
Kid Cuisine, with mini-franks	380	N.A.	N.A.	14	130	40
Kraft regular packaged dinner, ¾ cup prepared	290	N.A.	N.A.	13	120	N.A.
deluxe packaged dinner, ¾ cup	260	N.A.	N.A.	8	70	N.A.

*Less than 2% U.S. RDA

Sodium (mg)	Potassium (mg)	Protein (g)	Carbohy-drate (g)	Calcium (% U.S. RDA)	Iron (% U.S. RDA)	Vitamin A (% U.S. RDA)	Vitamin C (% U.S. RDA)
890	80	16	35	2	10	*	*
870	190	14	9	10	2	4	*
510	420	18	9	4	10	10	20
790	N.A.	8	30	4	10	8	10
280	380	12	40	4	10	6	2
850	N.A.	8	23	2	10	N.A.	N.A.
810	300	11	15	4	8	6	10
870	N.A.	11	48	10	15	10	10
930	N.A.	11	36	20	6	10	*
450	340	14	46	25	20	150	10
N.A.	N.A.	12	32	N.A.	N.A.	N.A.	N.A.
370	N.A.	9	23	15	6	6	*
960	N.A.	6	24	8	8	10	*
1110	N.A.	5	26	10	10	N.A.	N.A.
610	110	8	N.A.	40	N.A.	N.A.	N.A.
1000	320	9	55	10	15	*	10
530	N.A.	9	34	8	10	10	*
580	N.A.	11	36	10	10	8	*

～ DINNER

	Calories	Saturated fat (g)	Polyunsat-urated fat (g)	Total fat (g)	Calories from fat	Choles-terol (mg)
Stouffer's entree, ½ of 12-oz pkg	250	N.A.	N.A.	13	120	N.A.
Swanson homestyle entree	400	N.A.	N.A.	21	190	N.A.
3-compartment dinner	380	N.A.	N.A.	15	140	N.A.
Pot Pie	220	N.A.	N.A.	9	80	N.A.
Tyson Looney Tunes Meals, Tweety	280	N.A.	N.A.	8	70	N.A.
Manicotti						
Budget Gourmet, cheese with meat sauce	450	N.A.	N.A.	26	230	50
Healthy Choice entree, cheese	230	2	<1	4	35	20
Le Menu entree, cheese	410	N.A.	N.A.	20	180	N.A.
Weight Watchers entree, cheese	280	4	1	8	70	75
Manwich, Hunt, 1 sandwich prepared, all varieties	320	5	1	13	120	50
Chili Fixins, 1 cup prepared	290	5	<1	14	130	65
Meatballs with noodles and peppers, Budget Gourmet, Italian style	310	N.A.	N.A.	12	110	55
Meatball stew, Lean Cuisine entree	250	3	1	10	90	85
Meatballs, Swedish						
Armour Classics dinner	330	N.A.	N.A.	18	160	80
Armour Dining Light, with noodles	290	N.A.	N.A.	10	90	N.A.
Budget Gourmet, with noodles	600	N.A.	N.A.	39	350	140
Stouffer's entree, in gravy with parsley noodles	480	N.A.	N.A.	26	230	N.A.
Swanson homestyle entree	350	N.A.	N.A.	22	200	N.A.
Meat loaf						
Armour Classics dinner	360	N.A.	N.A.	17	150	65
Banquet dinner	440	N.A.	N.A.	27	240	85

*Less than 2% U.S. RDA

Sodium (mg)	Potassium (mg)	Protein (g)	Carbohydrate (g)	Calcium (% U.S. RDA)	Iron (% U.S. RDA)	Vitamin A (% U.S. RDA)	Vitamin C (% U.S. RDA)
730	140	12	22	25	2	2	*
980	N.A.	15	38	45	10	2	4
990	N.A.	12	49	20	15	70	8
880	N.A.	8	27	15	6	8	*
630	N.A.	10	42	N.A.	N.A.	N.A.	N.A.
920	N.A.	20	33	45	15	100	*
450	590	15	34	15	15	25	10
1030	N.A.	17	40	40	10	25	80
490	690	17	33	35	10	30	15
730	540	17	32	4	20	15	6
980	870	20	20	6	25	20	40
1120	N.A.	20	29	6	40	*	*
940	440	21	20	4	15	30	6
720	460	19	23	10	20	50	15
480	260	18	37	6	*	*	15
1090	N.A.	23	40	15	6	10	4
1510	350	24	37	6	15	2	2
780	N.A.	17	22	10	15	10	2
1170	590	20	32	6	20	8	20
770	900	26	27	6	25	30	40

～ DINNER

	Calories	Saturated fat (g)	Polyunsaturated fat (g)	Total fat (g)	Calories from fat	Cholesterol (mg)
Cookin' Bag, 4 oz	200	N.A.	N.A.	14	130	N.A.
Budget Gourmet Light & Healthy dinner, Italian style	270	4	2	10	90	45
Stouffer's homestyle dinner	410	N.A.	N.A.	22	200	N.A.
Swanson 4-compartment dinner	430	N.A.	N.A.	22	200	N.A.
Mexican-style dinner						
Banquet	490	N.A.	N.A.	18	160	N.A.
Combination	520	N.A.	N.A.	17	150	N.A.
Swanson Combination 4-compartment dinner	520	N.A.	N.A.	24	220	N.A.
Hungry Man	820	N.A.	N.A.	41	370	N.A.
Noodles and beef						
Banquet Family Entree, ¼ of 32-oz pkg	200	N.A.	N.A.	7	60	N.A.
Heinz, ½ of 15-oz can	170	N.A.	N.A.	8	70	N.A.
Noodles and chicken						
Banquet dinner	350	N.A.	N.A.	15	140	45
Heinz, ½ of 15-oz can	160	N.A.	N.A.	7	60	N.A.
Swanson 3-compartment dinner	260	N.A.	N.A.	9	80	N.A.
Noodles Romanoff, Stouffer's side dish, ⅓ of 12-oz pkg	170	N.A.	N.A.	9	80	N.A.
Noodle Roni, Golden Grain, ½ cup, all flavors	250	N.A.	N.A.	12	110	N.A.
1-step, ½ cup, all flavors	220	N.A.	N.A.	12	110	N.A.
Noodles and sauce, Lipton pouch, ½ cup, all varieties	200	N.A.	N.A.	9	80	N.A.
Noodles and tuna, Heinz, 1 cup canned	170	N.A.	N.A.	5	45	N.A.
Oven Stuffs, Quaker, all varieties	340	N.A.	N.A.	15	140	33
Oysters, breaded and fried, 6 medium	170	3	3	11	100	72

*Less than 2% U.S. RDA

Sodium (mg)	Potassium (mg)	Protein (g)	Carbohy-drate (g)	Calcium (% U.S. RDA)	Iron (% U.S. RDA)	Vitamin A (% U.S. RDA)	Vitamin C (% U.S. RDA)
N.A.	N.A.	10	8	N.A.	N.A.	N.A.	N.A.
480	570	20	30	10	15	100	60
1170	630	25	29	4	10	20	10
1030	N.A.	17	41	8	20	4	15
2000	430	18	62	10	20	8	15
1980	420	20	72	20	20	10	10
1580	N.A.	17	60	15	20	25	6
2080	N.A.	25	88	30	25	40	10
N.A.	N.A.	13	22	N.A.	N.A.	N.A.	N.A.
830	N.A.	8	17	2	10	N.A.	N.A.
460	250	10	42	2	15	140	4
930	N.A.	6	19	2	4	N.A.	N.A.
860	N.A.	11	35	4	10	8	10
840	100	7	15	8	4	2	*
630	180	7	27	8	8	8	*
670	160	6	24	6	6	10	6
550	N.A.	6	23	6	*	6	6
950	N.A.	11	20	2	6	N.A.	N.A.
530	180	20	31	25	20	15	*
370	220	8	10	6	40	*	N.A.

	Calories	Saturated fat (g)	Polyunsaturated fat (g)	Total fat (g)	Calories from fat	Cholesterol (mg)
Pasta Accents, Green Giant, ½ cup, all varieties	100	2	<1	5	45	5
Pasta alfredo, Budget Gourmet side dish	200	N.A.	N.A.	8	70	25
Pasta, angel hair, Weight Watchers entree	210	1	2	5	45	20
Pasta carbonara, Stouffer's side dish	620	N.A.	N.A.	45	410	N.A.
Pasta casino, Stouffer's side dish	300	N.A.	N.A.	10	90	N.A.
Pasta Dijon, Green Giant microwave garden gourmet, 9.5-oz pkg	260	9	1	17	150	55
pasta Florentine	230	5	1	9	80	25
Pasta Hearty Ones, Lipton microwave side dish, all varieties	340	N.A.	N.A.	4	35	7
Pasta Mexicali, Stouffer's side dish	490	N.A.	N.A.	31	280	N.A.
Oriental	300	N.A.	N.A.	14	130	N.A.
Pasta Parmesan, Green Giant, 5.5 oz	170	2	0	5	45	10
Pasta primavera						
Stouffer's side dish, ½ of 10⅝-oz pkg	270	N.A.	N.A.	21	190	N.A.
Weight Watchers entree	260	<1	3	11	100	5
Pasta rigati, Weight Watchers entree	300	2	1	9	80	25
Pasta salad, Fantastic Foods, ½ cup prepared, all varieties	180	N.A.	N.A.	10	90	N.A.
Pasta Trio, Tyson Gourmet Selection dinner	450	N.A.	N.A.	17	150	N.A.
Pierogis, Mrs. T's pasta pockets, 1 pierogi	60	N.A.	N.A.	<1	N.A.	3
Pizza, frozen						
Celeste, ¼ of large pizza	360	7	2	20	180	17

*Less than 2% U.S. RDA

Sodium (mg)	Potassium (mg)	Protein (g)	Carbohy-drate (g)	Calcium (% U.S. RDA)	Iron (% U.S. RDA)	Vitamin A (% U.S. RDA)	Vitamin C (% U.S. RDA)
250	125	4	12	4	6	45	25
390	N.A.	14	17	15	6	4	6
420	650	12	23	15	15	15	8
780	280	19	34	30	6	4	2
800	260	9	44	8	10	10	10
630	310	7	21	8	8	25	50
840	290	14	27	30	10	190	10
1240	620	15	62	10	15	25	8
1020	280	16	36	30	10	10	15
760	180	8	35	4	10	50	8
510	160	9	24	15	6	4	8
580	150	7	13	15	2	15	10
800	260	15	22	30	10	35	30
490	720	20	35	15	20	30	25
180	N.A.	4	19	N.A.	N.A.	N.A.	N.A.
890	N.A.	21	53	N.A.	N.A.	N.A.	N.A.
160	N.A.	2	11	*	2	*	*
920	280	15	29	25	8	20	*

	Calories	Saturated fat (g)	Polyunsaturated fat (g)	Total fat (g)	Calories from fat	Cholesterol (mg)
pizza for one	570	9	3	31	280	23
Kid Cuisine, cheese, 1 pkg	240	N.A.	N.A.	4	35	20
Lean Cuisine, French bread, 1 pkg	340	3	2	11	100	29
Stouffer's traditional, ½ pkg	360	N.A.	N.A.	18	160	N.A.
French bread, ½ pkg	410	N.A.	N.A.	19	170	N.A.
Weight Watchers, 1 serving, all varieties	320	4	2	9	80	33
French bread, 1 serving, all varieties	330	3	2	12	110	30
Pizza, hamburger, Tyson Looney Tunes Meals, Wile E. Coyote	300	N.A.	N.A.	12	110	N.A.
Pork chow mein Bi-Pack, La Choy, ¾ cup	80	1	<1	4	35	14
Pork, loin of, Swanson 4-compartment dinner	310	N.A.	N.A.	12	110	N.A.
Pork, sweet and sour, La Choy entree	250	1	<1	4	35	18
Pot Roast						
Armour Classics dinner, Yankee	310	N.A.	N.A.	12	110	85
Budget Gourmet Light & Healthy dinner, beef	210	2	1	8	70	65
Budget Gourmet 3-dish dinner, Yankee	380	N.A.	N.A.	21	190	70
Healthy Choice dinner, Yankee	260	2	<1	4	35	45
Le Menu dinner, Yankee	370	N.A.	N.A.	15	140	N.A.
Right Course, Homestyle	220	2	<1	7	60	35
Potato, baked, Weight Watchers entree, all varieties	280	2	1	6	50	35
Ravioli						
Budget Gourmet Slim Selects, cheese	260	N.A.	N.A.	7	60	45

*Less than 2% U.S. RDA

Sodium (mg)	Potassium (mg)	Protein (g)	Carbohy-drate (g)	Calcium (% U.S. RDA)	Iron (% U.S. RDA)	Vitamin A (% U.S. RDA)	Vitamin C (% U.S. RDA)
1320	410	22	50	40	10	25	*
390	390	10	41	20	15	10	8
900	340	20	40	30	20	6	15
740	220	16	33	20	10	6	6
1060	320	18	41	25	15	10	10
660	450	25	35	40	10	25	30
820	390	21	27	40	20	20	15
620	N.A.	10	37	N.A.	N.A.	N.A.	N.A.
950	275	5	7	2	4	15	20
770	N.A.	22	28	4	8	60	8
1540	215	6	48	2	8	15	6
670	710	25	26	4	20	70	20
440	580	23	19	4	10	100	15
690	N.A.	27	22	15	10	60	10
310	350	19	36	4	10	10	15
780	N.A.	27	31	4	20	140	15
550	480	17	22	2	8	50	8
670	820	18	39	20	10	25	30
960	N.A.	12	36	25	10	15	6

	Calories	Saturated fat (g)	Polyunsaturated fat (g)	Total fat (g)	Calories from fat	Cholesterol (mg)
Franco American, 1 cup canned, Beef RavioliOs	250	N.A.	N.A.	8	70	N.A.
hearty pasta beef, 1 cup canned	280	N.A.	N.A.	11	100	N.A.
Healthy Choice entree, cheese	240	1	<1	2	18	30
Kid Cuisine, mini-cheese, 1 pkg	250	N.A.	N.A.	2	18	20
Weight Watchers entree, cheese	290	4	1	9	80	85
Rice (see also Grains, Pasta & Flour)						
Rice and beans pouch, Lipton, ½ cup, all flavors	150	N.A.	N.A.	4	35	N.A.
Rice, Chinese fried, La Choy, ¾ cup	190	<1	<1	1	10	0
Rice, Minute microwave dishes, single size, ½ cup, all varieties	160	N.A.	N.A.	4	35	21
Rice pilaf						
Budget Gourmet side dish	240	N.A.	N.A.	9	80	10
Fantastic Foods quick brown, ½ cup, miso, Spanish	100	N.A.	N.A.	<1	N.A.	N.A.
Green Giant Rice Originals, ½ cup	110	<1	0	1	10	2
Rice-a-Roni, ½ cup, all flavors	140	N.A.	N.A.	4	35	N.A.
Savory Classics, ½ cup, all flavors	160	N.A.	N.A.	6	50	N.A.
Rice and sauce pouch, Lipton, ½ cup, all flavors	160	N.A.	N.A.	4	35	N.A.
Rigatoni						
Lean Cuisine entree, with meat sauce and cheese	260	3	1	10	90	40
Healthy Choice entree, with meat sauce	240	2	<1	4	35	20

*Less than 2% U.S. RDA

Sodium (mg)	Potassium (mg)	Protein (g)	Carbohydrate (g)	Calcium (% U.S. RDA)	Iron (% U.S. RDA)	Vitamin A (% U.S. RDA)	Vitamin C (% U.S. RDA)
920	N.A.	9	35	2	10	8	10
810	N.A.	9	35	4	6	15	10
460	590	15	40	25	15	50	8
730	460	6	52	8	15	10	10
630	720	18	34	35	15	35	15
470	N.A.	6	27	15	*	4	10
820	30	4	41	*	15	*	*
550	80	5	24	4	4	6	*
350	N.A.	4	35	4	4	4	4
250	N.A.	3	21	N.A.	N.A.	N.A.	N.A.
530	55	2	21	*	4	*	*
750	110	3	25	*	6	6	*
640	120	4	23	2	6	4	*
520	N.A.	3	26	4	*	*	8
870	530	18	25	20	10	20	10
470	700	16	36	20	20	35	8

	Calories	Saturated fat (g)	Polyunsaturated fat (g)	Total fat (g)	Calories from fat	Cholesterol (mg)
Scallops, breaded and fried, 6 large (3 oz)	210	2	3	10	90	57
Scallops and Shrimp Mariner, Budget Gourmet 3-dish dinner	320	N.A.	N.A.	9	80	70
Seafood with natural herbs, Armour Classics Lite dinner	190	N.A.	N.A.	2	18	35
Seafood creole with rice, Swanson homestyle entree	240	N.A.	N.A.	6	50	N.A.
Seafood linguini, Weight Watchers entree	210	1	1	7	60	5
Seafood Newburg						
Budget Gourmet entree	350	N.A.	N.A.	12	110	70
Healthy Choice entree	200	1	<1	3	25	55
Seafood platter, Mrs. Paul's	590	N.A.	N.A.	31	280	N.A.
Shells						
Budget Gourmet, shells and beef	340	N.A.	N.A.	14	130	35
Le Menu Light Style dinner, 3-cheese stuffed	280	4	1	8	70	25
Stouffer's dinner, cheese stuffed	310	N.A.	N.A.	14	130	N.A.
Stouffer's entree, shells and cheese, tomato sauce	330	N.A.	N.A.	15	140	N.A.
Shrimp, baby bay, Armour Classics Lite dinner	220	N.A.	N.A.	6	50	105
Shrimp, breaded and fried, 12 large (3 oz)	210	2	5	12	110	159
Shrimp Cajun style, Mrs. Paul's Light entree	200	N.A.	N.A.	3	25	N.A.
Shrimp and chicken Cantonese, Lean Cuisine entree	270	1	3	9	80	100
Shrimp chow mein Bi-Pack, La Choy, ¾ cup	70	<1	<1	1	10	19
Shrimp and clams with linguini, Mrs. Paul's Light entree	280	N.A.	N.A.	9	80	N.A.

*Less than 2% U.S. RDA

Sodium (mg)	Potassium (mg)	Protein (g)	Carbohy-drate (g)	Calcium (% U.S. RDA)	Iron (% U.S. RDA)	Vitamin A (% U.S. RDA)	Vitamin C (% U.S. RDA)
430	320	18	9	4	6	N.A.	N.A.
690	N.A.	16	43	15	4	15	20
1020	350	13	29	25	6	10	60
810	N.A.	7	40	10	8	15	50
750	140	11	27	2	6	8	15
660	N.A.	17	43	10	4	4	*
440	270	13	30	6	8	*	6
1220	N.A.	20	58	8	15	*	2
990	N.A.	20	34	25	10	100	4
710	N.A.	16	35	20	10	25	50
1050	550	16	29	35	10	15	10
850	450	17	32	35	6	6	10
890	260	12	31	15	15	15	15
320	200	18	9	6	6	N.A.	N.A.
860	N.A.	10	34	6	2	*	10
920	300	22	25	4	6	10	6
860	210	7	6	4	6	10	25
790	N.A.	13	38	4	10	*	*

～ DINNER

	Calories	Saturated fat (g)	Polyunsat- urated fat (g)	Total fat (g)	Calories from fat	Choles- terol (mg)
Shrimp creole						
Armour Classics Lite dinner	260	N.A.	N.A.	2	18	45
Healthy Choice dinner	230	<1	<1	2	18	60
Shrimp with fettucine, Budget Gourmet	630	N.A.	N.A.	20	180	145
Shrimp marinara, Healthy Choice dinner	260	<1	<1	1	10	55
Shrimp primavera						
Mrs. Paul's Light entree	180	1	1	3	25	N.A.
Right Course entree	240	1	1	7	60	50
Sirloin, chopped						
Le Menu dinner	440	N.A.	N.A.	25	230	N.A.
Swanson 4-compartment dinner	370	N.A.	N.A.	19	170	N.A.
Sirloin roast dinners						
Armour Classics	190	N.A.	N.A.	4	35	55
Budget Gourmet	560	N.A.	N.A.	14	130	85
Light & Healthy entree, wine sauce	230	2	1	6	50	30
Slim Selects, in herb sauce	290	N.A.	N.A.	12	110	25
Sirloin tips						
Armour Classics dinner	230	N.A.	N.A.	7	60	70
Budget Gourmet 3-dish dinner, in Burgundy sauce	310	N.A.	N.A.	11	100	65
Budget Gourmet, with country-style vegetables	310	N.A.	N.A.	18	160	40
Healthy Choice dinner	290	3	<1	6	50	70
Le Menu dinner	400	N.A.	N.A.	19	170	N.A.
Swanson homestyle entree, in Burgundy sauce	270	N.A.	N.A.	10	90	N.A.
Weight Watchers entree, with mushrooms in wine sauce	220	3	2	7	60	50
Sole, fillet of, Le Menu dinner	360	N.A.	N.A.	14	130	N.A.

*Less than 2% U.S. RDA

Sodium (mg)	Potassium (mg)	Protein (g)	Carbohy-drate (g)	Calcium (% U.S. RDA)	Iron (% U.S. RDA)	Vitamin A (% U.S. RDA)	Vitamin C (% U.S. RDA)
900	420	6	53	6	15	8	200
430	450	8	45	8	10	8	140
660	N.A.	10	38	10	15	20	8
320	320	10	51	6	15	10	190
840	N.A.	11	28	10	10	*	20
590	150	12	32	8	10	30	4
1030	N.A.	25	29	10	20	*	10
850	N.A.	21	29	8	15	110	8
970	500	19	21	6	15	60	30
700	N.A.	13	36	4	25	8	10
570	430	17	33	4	10	90	15
770	N.A.	19	27	6	15	8	4
820	560	22	20	10	15	45	20
720	N.A.	24	28	6	20	4	10
570	N.A.	16	21	6	2	15	4
350	540	25	33	2	15	70	70
780	N.A.	29	29	10	20	8	35
570	N.A.	17	27	2	15	8	*
540	160	20	19	2	10	10	6
940	N.A.	18	40	10	10	40	4

~ DINNER

	Calories	Saturated fat (g)	Polyunsaturated fat (g)	Total fat (g)	Calories from fat	Cholesterol (mg)
Sole au gratin, Healthy Choice dinner	270	N.A.	N.A.	5	45	55
Sole, Healthy Choice entree, lemon butter sauce	230	2	1	4	35	45
Sole, stuffed, Weight Watchers entree, Newburg sauce	310	1	2	9	80	5
Souper Combo, Campbell's, chicken soup combos	310	N.A.	N.A.	14	130	N.A.
all other combos	440	N.A.	N.A.	22	200	N.A.
Spaghetti						
Armour Dining Light dinner, with beef and mushroom sauce	220	N.A.	N.A.	8	70	20
Banquet dinner, with meatballs	290	N.A.	N.A.	10	90	30
Budget Gourmet, with Italian sausage	400	N.A.	N.A.	19	170	48
Franco American, ½ of 14¾-oz can, tomato sauce with cheese	190	N.A.	N.A.	2	18	N.A.
meatballs in tomato sauce	220	N.A.	N.A.	8	70	N.A.
Franco American SpaghettiOs, ½ of 15-oz can, tomato and cheese sauce	170	N.A.	N.A.	2	18	N.A.
meatballs or sliced beef franks in tomato sauce	220	N.A.	N.A.	9	80	N.A.
Healthy Choice entree, with meat sauce	280	2	2	4	35	15
Heinz, ½ of 15½-oz can, with cheese or meat	170	N.A.	N.A.	4	35	N.A.
Kid Cuisine entree, with meat sauce	310	N.A.	N.A.	12	110	35
Lean Cuisine entree, with beef and mushroom sauce	280	2	1	7	60	25

*Less than 2% U.S. RDA

Sodium (mg)	Potassium (mg)	Protein (g)	Carbohy-drate (g)	Calcium (% U.S. RDA)	Iron (% U.S. RDA)	Vitamin A (% U.S. RDA)	Vitamin C (% U.S. RDA)
470	420	16	40	8	6	*	10
390	380	16	33	6	4	*	*
940	670	19	38	10	10	10	20
1370	N.A.	15	31	4	10	10	*
1440	N.A.	16	44	20	15	20	15
440	570	12	25	8	15	20	20
580	540	11	44	4	20	170	25
770	N.A.	17	3	10	15	8	6
810	N.A.	5	36	2	6	8	*
850	N.A.	9	28	2	10	8	4
920	N.A.	4	34	2	6	10	*
970	N.A.	8	26	2	10	10	6
260	510	14	47	6	15	15	70
1040	N.A.	6	26	2	8	N.A.	N.A.
690	370	9	43	8	15	15	15
940	590	16	38	8	15	8	10

	Calories	Saturated fat (g)	Polyunsat-urated fat (g)	Total fat (g)	Calories from fat	Choles-terol (mg)
Snoopy's Choice entree, Healthy Choice for Kids, with meatballs and sauce	270	3	<1	5	45	35
Stouffer's entree, with meat sauce or meatballs	380	N.A.	N.A.	13	120	N.A.
Swanson homestyle entree, with Italian-style meatballs	460	N.A.	N.A.	19	170	N.A.
3-compartment dinner, with meatballs	370	N.A.	N.A.	16	140	N.A.
Tyson Looney Tunes Meals, with meatballs, Daffy Duck	300	N.A.	N.A.	8	70	N.A.
Weight Watchers entree, with meat sauce	280	3	1	7	60	25
Spanish rice, 1 cup canned	150	N.A.	N.A.	4	35	N.A.
Steak, chopped, Swanson Hungry Man dinner	640	N.A.	N.A.	37	330	N.A.
Steak Diane, Armour Classics Lite dinner	290	N.A.	N.A.	9	80	80
Steak, pepper						
Armour Classics Lite dinner	220	N.A.	N.A.	4	35	35
Budget Gourmet, with rice	300	N.A.	N.A.	9	80	25
Healthy Choice dinner	290	3	<1	6	50	65
entree	200	2	<1	3	25	30
La Choy Dinner Classics, ¾ cup prepared	180	3	2	9	80	60
Le Menu dinner	370	N.A.	N.A.	13	120	N.A.
Stouffer's entree, green pepper with rice	330	N.A.	N.A.	11	100	N.A.
Tyson Gourmet Selection dinner	330	N.A.	N.A.	11	100	N.A.
Steak, Salisbury						
Armour Classics dinner	350	N.A.	N.A.	17	150	55
parmigiana	410	N.A.	N.A.	21	190	60
Armour Classics Lite dinner	300	N.A.	N.A.	11	100	40

*Less than 2% U.S. RDA

Sodium (mg)	Potassium (mg)	Protein (g)	Carbohy-drate (g)	Calcium (% U.S. RDA)	Iron (% U.S. RDA)	Vitamin A (% U.S. RDA)	Vitamin C (% U.S. RDA)
370	470	15	41	4	10	20	4
1510	690	19	46	10	15	20	10
1010	N.A.	16	56	15	40	20	35
1010	N.A.	12	45	10	15	20	20
820	N.A.	12	46	N.A.	N.A.	N.A.	N.A.
610	560	20	32	8	20	40	45
1040	220	3	28	4	10	15	8
1600	N.A.	35	41	6	30	8	15
440	820	27	25	4	25	60	20
970	320	17	29	6	15	10	25
800	N.A.	15	39	4	4	6	4
530	380	24	34	4	10	8	120
300	200	14	29	2	8	4	30
760	490	17	9	2	10	30	*
1030	N.A.	25	38	4	20	20	20
1440	410	21	36	2	10	4	10
1130	N.A.	20	38	N.A.	N.A.	N.A.	N.A.
1430	530	22	26	10	25	6	40
1120	540	22	32	15	25	8	15
980	660	21	29	10	25	6	25

	Calories	Saturated fat (g)	Polyunsaturated fat (g)	Total fat (g)	Calories from fat	Cholesterol (mg)
Armour Dining Light, with vegetables, Italian sauce	200	N.A.	N.A.	8	70	55
Banquet dinner	500	N.A.	N.A.	34	310	80
Extra Helping dinner	910	N.A.	N.A.	60	540	175
Banquet Family Entree, ¼ of 32-oz pkg	300	N.A.	N.A.	22	200	N.A.
Budget Gourmet 3-dish dinner, sirloin	410	N.A.	N.A.	22	200	105
Light & Healthy entree	260	4	1	9	80	30
Slim Selects entree	280	N.A.	N.A.	8	70	75
Healthy Choice dinner	300	3	<1	7	60	50
Le Menu Light style dinner	220	4	1	7	60	45
Lean Cuisine, with Italian sauce and vegetables	280	5	1	15	140	100
Stouffer's entree	250	N.A.	N.A.	14	130	N.A.
Stouffer's dinner, with gravy and mushrooms	400	N.A.	N.A.	23	210	N.A.
Swanson 4-compartment dinner	410	N.A.	N.A.	18	160	N.A.
Homestyle entree	480	N.A.	N.A.	34	310	N.A.
Hungry Man dinner	680	N.A.	N.A.	41	370	N.A.
Tyson Gourmet Selection dinner	430	N.A.	N.A.	26	230	N.A.
Weight Watchers entree, Romana	190	2	1	7	60	40
Steak, Swiss						
Budget Gourmet 3-dish dinner	450	N.A.	N.A.	22	200	70
Swanson 4-compartment dinner	340	N.A.	N.A.	11	100	N.A.
Stew, canned beef with vegetables, 1 cup	190	N.A.	N.A.	7	60	33
Suddenly Salad, Betty Crocker pkg mix, ⅙ of pkg, all varieties	180	N.A.	N.A.	8	70	N.A.

*Less than 2% U.S. RDA

Sodium (mg)	Potassium (mg)	Protein (g)	Carbohy-drate (g)	Calcium (% U.S. RDA)	Iron (% U.S. RDA)	Vitamin A (% U.S. RDA)	Vitamin C (% U.S. RDA)
1000	650	18	14	6	20	10	4
600	590	23	26	4	20	10	10
740	1020	50	49	8	45	15	15
N.A.	N.A.	13	12	N.A.	N.A.	N.A.	N.A.
890	N.A.	26	28	20	15	20	10
510	620	21	28	8	10	70	30
870	N.A.	21	31	8	35	20	6
480	610	19	41	6	15	2	120
830	N.A.	18	21	8	15	4	*
840	700	25	12	15	15	10	10
1070	380	21	9	2	15	30	10
1230	550	25	24	15	20	15	10
880	N.A.	19	43	6	15	4	6
1170	N.A.	22	22	25	15	*	2
1730	N.A.	41	37	30	35	8	10
810	N.A.	16	34	N.A.	N.A.	N.A.	N.A.
470	480	20	13	10	15	25	25
1110	N.A.	23	40	10	4	4	25
740	N.A.	23	38	6	25	8	15
970	410	14	17	4	10	45	10
390	115	4	21	2	6	6	*

	Calories	Saturated fat (g)	Polyunsaturated fat (g)	Total fat (g)	Calories from fat	Cholesterol (mg)
Sweet and sour dinner classics, La Choy, ¾ cup	310	1	3	6	50	50
Tamales with sauce (Van Camp's), 1 cup canned	290	N.A.	N.A.	16	140	N.A.
Tortellini						
Birds Eye for One, 5.5 oz, cheese	210	N.A.	N.A.	5	45	30
Budget Gourmet side dish, cheese	180	N.A.	N.A.	6	50	15
Green Giant, 5.5 oz, cheese marinara	260	N.A.	N.A.	9	80	N.A.
microwave garden gourmet, 9.5-oz pkg, Provencale	210	1	1	5	45	15
Stouffer's entree, beef with marinara sauce	360	N.A.	N.A.	12	110	N.A.
Stouffer's entree, cheese in alfredo sauce	600	N.A.	N.A.	40	360	N.A.
with tomato sauce	360	N.A.	N.A.	16	140	N.A.
with vinaigrette dressing	400	N.A.	N.A.	27	240	N.A.
Weight Watches entree, cheese	310	1	1	6	50	15
Tortilla Grande, Stouffer's entree	530	N.A.	N.A.	33	300	N.A.
Tuna Helper, General Mills, ⅕ pkg prepared, all varieties except pot pie, salad	250	N.A.	N.A.	10	90	N.A.
tuna pot pie (⅙ pkg), tuna salad (⅕ pkg)	420	N.A.	N.A.	27	240	N.A.
Tuna noodle casserole, Stouffer's entree	310	N.A.	N.A.	13	120	N.A.
Tuna pasta casserole, Mrs. Paul's Light entree	270	N.A.	N.A.	7	60	N.A.
Tuna Pie, Banquet	540	N.A.	N.A.	33	300	30
Turkey						
Armour Classics dinner, dressing and gravy	320	N.A.	N.A.	12	110	50

*Less than 2% U.S. RDA

Sodium (mg)	Potassium (mg)	Protein (g)	Carbohy-drate (g)	Calcium (% U.S. RDA)	Iron (% U.S. RDA)	Vitamin A (% U.S. RDA)	Vitamin C (% U.S. RDA)
960	360	32	31	4	15	60	8
1130	240	8	29	4	20	40	N.A.
500	320	11	31	10	10	20	20
400	N.A.	7	25	10	8	4	4
930	310	8	37	10	8	25	8
720	550	7	36	8	8	150	4
780	580	18	45	10	15	10	10
930	270	28	32	50	8	4	6
860	420	18	37	30	8	20	10
540	190	15	24	25	6	35	45
570	510	14	50	20	15	20	25
910	730	24	34	40	15	20	15
930	250	15	29	6	6	8	*
880	220	14	30	2	10	8	*
1340	350	17	31	15	6	2	*
960	N.A.	22	29	30	8	2	6
810	280	17	44	15	15	10	4
1280	520	19	34	10	15	60	15

∾ DINNER

	Calories	Saturated fat (g)	Polyunsat- urated fat (g)	Total fat (g)	Calories from fat	Choles- terol (mg)
Banquet Cookin' Bag, 5 oz, with gravy	100	N.A.	N.A.	6	50	N.A.
Banquet dinner	390	N.A.	N.A.	20	180	40
Extra Helping dinner	750	N.A.	N.A.	42	380	65
Budget Gourmet 3-dish dinner, breast	290	N.A.	N.A.	9	80	45
breast Dijon	340	N.A.	N.A.	12	110	65
Slim Selects, glazed	270	N.A.	N.A.	5	45	50
Healthy Choice dinner, breast	290	2	1	5	45	45
Le Menu dinner, breast, with mushroom gravy	270	N.A.	N.A.	6	50	N.A.
Stouffer's dinner, roast breast	330	N.A.	N.A.	10	90	N.A.
Swanson 4-compartment dinner	350	N.A.	N.A.	11	100	N.A.
homestyle entree, dress- ing and potatoes	290	N.A.	N.A.	13	120	N.A.
Hungry Man dinner	550	N.A.	N.A.	18	160	N.A.
Turkey breast						
Budget Gourmet Light & Healthy dinner, stuffed	230	2	2	6	50	40
Lean Cuisine entree, mushroom sauce	240	2	1	7	60	50
Weight Watchers entree, stuffed	260	4	1	10	90	80
Turkey casserole, Stouffer's entree, gravy and dressing	360	N.A.	N.A.	17	150	N.A.
Turkey Dijon, Lean Cuisine entree	270	3	1	10	90	60
Turkey divan, Le Menu Light style dinner	280	4	1	9	80	40
Turkey à la king, Budget Gourmet, with rice	390	N.A.	N.A.	18	160	75
Turkey in mild curry sauce, Right Course, with rice pilaf	320	2	1	8	70	50

*Less than 2% U.S. RDA

Sodium (mg)	Potassium (mg)	Protein (g)	Carbohy-drate (g)	Calcium (% U.S. RDA)	Iron (% U.S. RDA)	Vitamin A (% U.S. RDA)	Vitamin C (% U.S. RDA)
N.A.	N.A.	7	5	N.A.	N.A.	N.A.	N.A.
1110	500	18	35	4	6	10	10
1980	880	29	68	10	20	15	15
1200	N.A.	16	36	4	10	4	10
860	N.A.	20	37	8	10	45	15
760	N.A.	17	39	2	6	*	4
420	540	21	39	4	10	4	80
1020	N.A.	17	37	4	10	50	15
1290	480	27	32	6	15	20	15
1110	N.A.	20	42	4	15	6	6
1020	N.A.	17	30	2	10	*	4
1810	N.A.	36	61	8	25	8	15
520	560	22	29	6	8	60	100
790	350	23	20	2	4	10	4
910	400	20	24	6	10	15	20
1090	250	23	29	10	10	4	*
900	470	24	22	15	6	50	2
840	N.A.	22	26	10	8	8	20
740	N.A.	20	36	15	6	10	4
570	550	23	40	10	8	10	10

～ DINNER

	Calories	Saturated fat (g)	Polyunsaturated fat (g)	Total fat (g)	Calories from fat	Cholesterol (mg)
Turkey pie						
Banquet	510	N.A.	N.A.	31	280	40
microwave, single crust	430	N.A.	N.A.	27	240	35
Stouffer's entree	540	N.A.	N.A.	36	320	N.A.
Swanson Pot Pie	390	N.A.	N.A.	22	200	N.A.
Hungry Man	750	N.A.	N.A.	42	380	N.A.
Turkey, roasted, Healthy Choice entree, mushrooms in gravy	200	1	1	3	25	25
Turkey tetrazzini, Stouffer's entree	380	N.A.	N.A.	20	180	N.A.
Veal marsala, Le Menu Light Style dinner	260	3	1	6	50	100
Veal parmigiana						
Armour Classics dinner	400	N.A.	N.A.	22	200	55
Banquet Cookin' Bag, 4 oz	230	N.A.	N.A.	11	100	N.A.
Budget Gourmet 3-dish dinner	440	N.A.	N.A.	20	180	165

*Less than 2% U.S. RDA

Sodium (mg)	Potassium (mg)	Protein (g)	Carbohy-drate (g)	Calcium (% U.S. RDA)	Iron (% U.S. RDA)	Vitamin A (% U.S. RDA)	Vitamin C (% U.S. RDA)
860	230	16	39	4	15	6	*
740	250	15	30	4	15	15	4
1300	260	20	35	10	10	25	*
720	N.A.	10	38	2	8	35	2
1670	N.A.	27	65	4	20	70	6
310	260	N.A.	N.A.	N.A.	N.A.	N.A.	N.A.
1170	300	22	28	10	8	2	*
820	N.A.	20	31	2	10	25	6
1320	520	18	34	15	20	20	45
N.A.	N.A.	10	20	N.A.	N.A.	N.A.	N.A.
1160	N.A.	26	39	30	25	100	10

~ FAST FOOD

~ *This information comes directly from the companies listed and is up-to-date at this writing. Several of the restaurants provide salad bars. To avoid duplication, Wendy's Salad Spot has been used as a typical fast-food salad bar; it is listed separately from the main Wendy's section, under Salad Bar. The salad dressings in that section are also found in "Fats, Oils, Margarines & Salad Dressings."*

Values for sugar and fiber content are not widely available and so are not included here. Some chains also do not provide information on saturated fat, polyunsaturated fat, or potassium.

ARBY'S/ BURGER KING

	Calories	Saturated fat (g)	Polyunsaturated fat (g)	Total fat (g)	Calories from fat	Cholesterol (mg)
Beef						
Beef 'n Cheddar	460	8	7	27	240	63
roast beef, regular	350	7	2	15	140	39
roast beef, super	500	9	5	22	200	40
Chicken						
chicken breast sandwich	490	5	10	25	230	91
roast chicken club	610	8	14	33	300	80
French fries	250	3	5	13	120	0
Ham 'n Cheese	290	5	6	14	130	45
Jamocha shake	370	3	2	11	100	35
Potato cakes	200	2	4	12	110	0
Turkey deluxe	380	4	8	17	150	39
Apple pie	310	4	1	14	130	4
Breakfast items						
bagel	270	1	3	6	50	29
with cream cheese	370	6	3	16	140	58
bagel sandwich, with egg and cheese	410	5	4	16	140	247
with bacon, egg, and cheese	450	7	4	20	180	252
with ham, egg, and cheese	440	6	4	17	150	266
with sausage, egg, and cheese	630	12	6	36	320	293
biscuit	330	3	2	17	150	2
with bacon	380	5	2	20	180	8
with bacon and egg	470	7	4	27	240	213
with sausage	480	8	4	29	260	33
with sausage and egg	570	10	5	36	320	240
croissant	180	2	1	10	90	4
with bacon, egg, and cheese	360	8	3	24	220	227
with egg and cheese	320	7	2	20	180	222

*Less than 2% U.S. RDA

Sodium (mg)	Potassium (mg)	Protein (g)	Carbohy-drate (g)	Calcium (% U.S. RDA)	Iron (% U.S. RDA)	Vitamin A (% U.S. RDA)	Vitamin C (% U.S. RDA)
960	360	26	28	6	20	8	*
590	370	22	32	8	20	*	2
800	500	25	50	10	25	15	60
1020	330	23	48	8	20	*	8
1500	430	31	40	15	20	*	*
115	240	2	30	*	6	*	*
1350	310	23	19	20	15	5	*
260	530	9	59	25	15	6	4
400	290	2	20	*	8	*	35
1050	350	24	33	8	15	6	8
410	N.A.	3	44	*	8	*	8
440	N.A.	10	44	*	10	*	*
520	N.A.	12	45	4	10	8	*
760	N.A.	19	46	15	15	10	*
870	N.A.	21	46	15	15	10	*
1110	N.A.	25	46	15	15	10	*
1140	N.A.	27	49	15	20	10	*
750	N.A.	5	42	20	15	*	*
870	N.A.	8	42	20	*	*	*
1030	N.A.	14	43	25	6	8	*
1010	N.A.	11	44	20	4	*	*
1170	N.A.	17	45	25	8	8	*
290	N.A.	4	18	4	6	*	*
720	N.A.	15	19	15	10	10	*
610	N.A.	13	19	15	10	10	*

~ BURGER KING

	Calories	Saturated fat (g)	Polyunsat-urated fat (g)	Total fat (g)	Calories from fat	Choles-terol (mg)
with ham, egg, and cheese	350	7	2	21	190	240
with sausage, egg, and cheese	530	13	5	40	360	268
danish (typical)	500	23	N.A.	36	320	6
French toast sticks	540	5	11	32	290	80
hash browns	210	3	3	12	110	3
scrambled egg platter	550	9	6	34	310	365
with bacon	610	11	7	39	350	373
with sausage	770	15	8	53	480	412
Burgers						
cheeseburger	320	7	1	15	140	50
deluxe	390	8	7	23	210	56
double cheeseburger	480	13	2	27	240	100
bacon double cheese-burger	520	14	2	31	280	105
deluxe	590	16	8	39	350	111
hamburger	270	4	1	11	100	37
Deluxe	340	6	7	19	170	43
Whopper	610	12	13	36	320	90
with cheese	710	16	13	44	400	115
Double Whopper	840	19	13	53	480	169
with cheese	940	24	14	61	550	194
Chicken						
BK broiler chicken sandwich	380	3	8	18	160	53
chicken sandwich	690	8	20	40	360	82
chicken tenders, 6 pc	240	3	3	13	120	46
Fish tenders	270	3	4	16	140	28
French fries, medium salted	340	10	<1	20	180	21
Milk shake						
chocolate	330	6	0	10	90	31

*Less than 2% U.S. RDA

Sodium (mg)	Potassium (mg)	Protein (g)	Carbohy-drate (g)	Calcium (% U.S. RDA)	Iron (% U.S. RDA)	Vitamin A (% U.S. RDA)	Vitamin C (% U.S. RDA)
960	N.A.	19	19	15	10	10	*
990	N.A.	21	22	15	15	10	*
290	N.A.	5	40	10	10	N.A.	N.A.
540	N.A.	10	53	8	15	*	*
320	N.A.	2	25	*	2	10	10
890	N.A.	17	44	10	15	20	10
1040	N.A.	21	44	10	15	20	10
1270	N.A.	26	47	10	20	20	10
660	N.A.	17	28	10	15	8	6
650	N.A.	18	29	10	15	10	10
850	N.A.	30	29	20	20	10	6
750	N.A.	32	26	20	20	8	*
800	N.A.	33	28	20	20	10	6
510	N.A.	15	28	4	15	4	6
500	N.A.	15	28	4	15	6	10
870	N.A.	27	45	8	25	10	20
1180	N.A.	32	47	20	25	20	20
930	N.A.	46	45	10	40	10	20
1250	N.A.	51	47	25	40	20	20
760	N.A.	24	31	6	15	8	10
1420	N.A.	26	56	8	20	4	*
540	N.A.	16	14	*	4	*	*
870	N.A.	12	18	4	6	*	*
240	N.A.	4	36	2	4	*	25
200	N.A.	9	49	30	4	8	4

∼ BURGER KING/ DAIRY QUEEN	Calories	Saturated fat (g)	Polyunsat- urated fat (g)	Total fat (g)	Calories from fat	Choles- terol (mg)
syrup added	410	6	0	11	100	33
strawberry, syrup added	390	6	0	10	90	33
vanilla	330	6	0	10	90	33
Ocean Catch Fish Filet	500	4	13	25	230	57
Onion rings	300	4	4	17	150	3
Salads (without dressing)						
chef	180	4	1	9	80	103
chunky chicken	140	1	1	4	35	49
garden	100	3	0	5	45	15
side	25	0	0	0	0	0
Brazier						
Burgers						
single hamburger	360	N.A.	N.A.	16	140	45
with cheese	410	N.A.	N.A.	20	180	50
double hamburger	530	N.A.	N.A.	28	250	85
with cheese	650	N.A.	N.A.	37	330	95
triple hamburger	710	N.A.	N.A.	45	410	135
with cheese	820	N.A.	N.A.	50	450	145
chicken sandwich	670	N.A.	N.A.	41	370	75
fish sandwich	400	N.A.	N.A.	17	150	50
with cheese	440	N.A.	N.A.	21	190	60
French fries, regular	200	N.A.	N.A.	10	90	10
large	320	N.A.	N.A.	16	140	15
Hot dog						
regular	280	N.A.	N.A.	16	140	45
with chili	320	N.A.	N.A.	20	180	55
with cheese	330	N.A.	N.A.	21	190	55
super	520	N.A.	N.A.	27	240	80
with chili	570	N.A.	N.A.	32	290	100
with cheese	580	N.A.	N.A.	34	310	100
Onion rings	280	N.A.	N.A.	16	140	15

*Less than 2% U.S. RDA

Sodium (mg)	Potassium (mg)	Protein (g)	Carbohy-drate (g)	Calcium (% U.S. RDA)	Iron (% U.S. RDA)	Vitamin A (% U.S. RDA)	Vitamin C (% U.S. RDA)
250	N.A.	10	68	30	*	*	*
230	N.A.	9	66	30	*	*	*
210	N.A.	9	51	30	*	*	*
880	N.A.	20	49	6	15	*	4
560	N.A.	4	34	10	4	15	*
570	N.A.	17	7	15	10	100	25
440	N.A.	20	8	4	8	90	35
125	N.A.	6	8	15	6	100	60
25	N.A.	1	5	4	4	90	20
630	N.A.	21	33	10	20	2	*
790	N.A.	24	33	20	20	4	*
660	N.A.	36	33	10	35	2	*
980	N.A.	43	34	35	35	8	*
690	N.A.	51	33	10	50	4	*
1010	N.A.	58	34	35	50	8	*
870	N.A.	29	46	*	2	*	15
880	N.A.	20	41	6	4	*	*
1040	N.A.	24	39	15	2	2	*
115	N.A.	2	25	*	6	*	25
190	N.A.	3	40	2	4	*	4
830	N.A.	11	21	8	8	*	*
990	N.A.	13	23	8	10	*	*
990	N.A.	15	21	15	8	2	*
1370	N.A.	17	44	15	15	*	*
1600	N.A.	21	47	15	15	*	*
1600	N.A.	22	45	25	8	2	*
140	N.A.	4	31	10	25	*	*

～ DAIRY QUEEN	Calories	Saturated fat (g)	Polyunsaturated fat (g)	Total fat (g)	Calories from fat	Cholesterol (mg)
Desserts						
banana split	540	N.A.	N.A.	11	100	30
Buster Bar	460	N.A.	N.A.	29	260	10
cone, small	140	N.A.	N.A.	4	35	10
regular	240	N.A.	N.A.	7	60	15
large	340	N.A.	N.A.	10	90	25
dipped cone, chocolate, small	190	N.A.	N.A.	9	80	10
regular	340	N.A.	N.A.	16	140	20
large	510	N.A.	N.A.	24	220	30
Dilly Bar	210	N.A.	N.A.	13	120	10
Double Delight	490	N.A.	N.A.	20	180	25
DQ Sandwich	140	N.A.	N.A.	4	35	5
float	410	N.A.	N.A.	7	60	20
freeze	500	N.A.	N.A.	12	110	30
Hot Fudge Brownie Delight	600	N.A.	N.A.	25	230	20
malt, chocolate, small	520	N.A.	N.A.	13	120	35
regular	760	N.A.	N.A.	18	160	50
large	1060	N.A.	N.A.	25	230	70
Mr. Misty, small	190	0	0	0	0	0
regular	250	0	0	0	0	0
large	340	0	0	0	0	0
Mr. Misty float	390	N.A.	N.A.	7	60	20
Mr. Misty freeze	500	N.A.	N.A.	12	110	30
Mr. Misty Kiss	70	0	0	0	0	0
parfait	430	N.A.	N.A.	8	70	30
Peanut Buster Parfait	740	N.A.	N.A.	34	310	30
shake, chocolate, small	490	N.A.	N.A.	13	120	35
regular	710	N.A.	N.A.	19	170	50
large	990	N.A.	N.A.	26	230	70
strawberry shortcake	540	N.A.	N.A.	11	100	25

*Less than 2% U.S. RDA

Sodium (mg)	Potassium (mg)	Protein (g)	Carbohydrate (g)	Calcium (% U.S. RDA)	Iron (% U.S. RDA)	Vitamin A (% U.S. RDA)	Vitamin C (% U.S. RDA)
150	N.A.	9	103	25	10	15	25
180	N.A.	10	41	10	6	2	*
45	N.A.	3	22	10	2	2	*
80	N.A.	6	38	15	4	4	*
115	N.A.	9	57	25	8	8	*
55	N.A.	3	25	10	2	2	*
100	N.A.	6	42	15	4	4	*
150	N.A.	9	64	25	8	8	*
50	N.A.	3	21	10	2	2	*
150	N.A.	9	69	20	8	6	*
40	N.A.	3	24	6	*	*	*
85	N.A.	5	82	20	6	4	*
180	N.A.	9	89	30	10	8	*
230	N.A.	9	85	20	10	6	*
180	N.A.	10	91	35	15	10	*
260	N.A.	14	134	45	25	15	*
360	N.A.	20	187	70	30	20	*
5	N.A.	0	48	*	*	*	*
5	N.A.	0	63	*	*	*	*
5	N.A.	0	84	*	*	*	*
95	N.A.	5	74	20	4	4	*
140	N.A.	9	91	30	8	8	*
5	N.A.	0	17	*	*	*	*
140	N.A.	8	76	25	8	8	6
250	N.A.	16	94	25	10	6	*
180	N.A.	10	82	35	10	10	*
260	N.A.	14	120	45	15	15	*
360	N.A.	19	168	70	20	20	*
220	N.A.	10	100	25	10	8	20

~ DIARY QUEEN/ KFC/ LONG JOHN SILVER'S	Calories	Saturated fat (g)	Polyunsaturated fat (g)	Total fat (g)	Calories from fat	Cholesterol (mg)
Sundae, chocolate, small	190	N.A.	N.A.	4	35	10
regular	310	N.A.	N.A.	8	70	20
large	440	N.A.	N.A.	10	90	30
Buttermilk biscuit, 1	240	3	2	12	110	1
Chicken Littles Sandwich	170	2	3	10	90	18
Cole slaw, 1 serving	120	1	3	7	60	5
Colonel's chicken sandwich	480	6	9	27	240	47
Corn on the cob, 1 ear	180	<1	2	3	25	<1
Extra Tasty Crispy Chicken, wing	250	4	3	19	170	67
breast, center	340	5	2	20	180	114
breast, side	340	6	2	22	200	81
drumstick	200	3	2	14	130	71
thigh	410	8	4	30	270	129
French fries	240	3	<1	12	110	2
Kentucky Nuggets, 1	45	<1	<1	3	25	12
Mashed potatoes and gravy	70	<1	<1	2	18	<1
Original Recipe Chicken, wing	180	3	2	12	110	65
breast, center	280	4	2	15	140	95
breast, side	270	4	2	17	150	75
drumstick	150	2	1	9	80	65
thigh	290	5	3	20	180	120
Catfish fillet, 1 pc	180	3	<1	11	100	25
Catfish fillet dinner (2 fillets, fries, slaw, 2 hush puppies)	860	10	6	42	380	65
Clam chowder with cod, 1 order	140	2	2	6	50	20
Clam dinner (clams, fries, slaw, 2 hush puppies)	980	10	6	45	410	15
Clams, breaded, 1 order	240	3	<1	12	110	3
Chicken Plank, 1 piece	110	1	<1	6	50	15

*Less than 2% U.S. RDA

Sodium (mg)	Potassium (mg)	Protein (g)	Carbohy- drate (g)	Calcium (% U.S. RDA)	Iron (% U.S. RDA)	Vitamin A (% U.S. RDA)	Vitamin C (% U.S. RDA)
75	N.A.	3	33	10	2	2	*
120	N.A.	5	56	20	6	4	*
170	N.A.	8	78	25	8	8	*
660	N.A.	5	28	10	10	*	*
330	N.A.	6	14	2	10	*	*
200	N.A.	2	13	4	*	6	35
1060	N.A.	21	39	4	8	*	*
20	N.A.	5	32	*	6	6	4
420	N.A.	12	9	2	4	*	*
790	N.A.	33	12	4	6	*	*
750	N.A.	22	14	4	6	*	*
320	N.A.	14	6	*	4	*	*
690	N.A.	20	14	4	8	2	*
140	N.A.	3	31	*	4	*	25
140	N.A.	3	2	*	*	*	*
340	N.A.	2	12	2	2	*	*
370	N.A.	12	6	4	8	*	*
670	N.A.	28	9	4	6	*	*
740	N.A.	19	11	6	8	*	*
280	N.A.	13	4	2	8	*	*
620	N.A.	18	11	6	8	2	*
310	230	10	10	*	35	4	*
990	1180	28	90	25	80	15	2
590	380	11	10	20	10	15	*
1200	870	21	122	30	25	4	2
410	80	7	26	4	6	*	*
320	150	8	6	2	4	*	*

~ LONG JOHN SILVER'S

	Calories	Saturated fat (g)	Polyunsat-urated fat (g)	Total fat (g)	Calories from fat	Choles-terol (mg)
Chicken Plank Dinner, 3 pc (3 planks, fries, slaw, 2 hush puppies)	830	9	5	39	350	55
Children's meals						
1 fish, fries, 1 hush puppy	440	5	<1	20	180	30
2 chicken planks, fries, 1 hush puppy	510	6	<1	24	220	30
1 fish, 1 chicken plank, fries, 1 hush puppy	550	6	1	26	230	45
Cole slaw, drained on fork, 1 order	140	1	4	6	50	15
Corn on the cob, 1 ear	270	3	4	14	130	3
Fish, battered, 1 pc	150	2	<1	8	70	30
Fish, homestyle, 1 pc	130	2	<1	7	60	20
Fish dinner, 3 pc (3 fish, fries, slaw, 2 hush puppies)	960	10	5	44	400	100
Fish and chicken dinner (1 fish, 2 chicken planks, fries, slaw, 2 hush puppies)	870	9	5	40	360	70
Fish and fries, 2 pc (2 fish, fries, 2 hush puppies)	660	7	1	30	270	60
Fish sandwich, homestyle	510	5	3	22	200	45
Fries, 1 order	220	3	<1	10	90	3
Gumbo with cod and shrimp, 1 order	120	2	3	8	70	25
Hush puppy, 1	70	<1	<1	2	18	3
Pie, lemon meringue, 1 slice	260	3	1	7	60	3
Pie, pecan, 1 slice	530	7	2	25	230	70
Salad, garden	170	N.A.	N.A.	9	80	3
Salad, ocean chef	250	<1	<1	9	80	80
Salad, seafood, 1 scoop	210	<1	3	5	45	90
Salad, side	20	N.A.	N.A.	N.A.	N.A.	0
Seafood platter (1 fish, 2 battered shrimp, clams, fries, slaw, 2 hush puppies)	970	10	6	46	410	70

*Less than 2% U.S. RDA

Sodium (mg)	Potassium (mg)	Protein (g)	Carbohy-drate (g)	Calcium (% U.S. RDA)	Iron (% U.S. RDA)	Vitamin A (% U.S. RDA)	Vitamin C (% U.S. RDA)
1340	1170	31	88	25	30	4	2
590	730	16	49	15	10	*	*
730	760	20	52	15	15	*	*
910	880	24	55	15	15	*	*
260	190	1	20	6	4	4	*
95	5	6	38	*	6	15	25
510	270	12	9	6	2	*	*
200	160	7	9	*	45	2	*
1890	1540	43	97	35	20	4	4
1520	1290	35	91	30	25	4	2
1120	1070	30	68	25	15	*	2
780	470	22	58	15	100	6	2
60	390	3	30	6	4	*	*
740	310	9	4	10	10	20	*
25	65	2	10	4	4	*	*
270	100	2	47	8	6	*	*
470	100	6	70	15	6	10	*
380	20	9	13	30	10	35	40
1340	160	24	19	35	40	50	25
570	100	14	26	15	20	25	*
20	N.A.	1	5	N.A.	2	20	4
1540	1100	30	109	35	25	4	2

~ LONG JOHN SILVER'S/ MCDONALD'S	Calories	Saturated fat (g)	Polyunsaturated fat (g)	Total fat (g)	Calories from fat	Cholesterol (mg)
Shrimp, battered, 1 pc	40	<1	<1	3	25	10
Shrimp, breaded, 1 order	190	2	<1	10	90	40
Shrimp dinner, battered, 6 pc (6 shrimp, fries, slaw, 2 hush puppies)	740	8	5	37	330	90
Shrimp and fish dinner (1 fish, 3 battered shrimp, fries, slaw, 2 hush puppies)	770	8	5	37	330	80
Shrimp, fish, and chicken dinner (2 battered shrimp, 1 fish, 1 chicken plank, fries, slaw, 2 hush puppies)	840	9	5	40	360	80
Vegetables, mixed, 1 order	60	<1	<1	2	18	0
Breakfast Items						
apple bran muffin	190	0	0	0	0	0
biscuit, with spread	260	3	<1	13	120	1
with bacon, egg, and cheese	440	8	2	26	230	253
with sausage	440	9	3	29	260	49
with sausage and egg	520	11	3	35	320	275
Cheerios, 1 box (⅔ oz)	80	<1	<1	1	10	0
danish, all varieties	410	4	2	19	170	33
eggs, scrambled	140	3	1	10	90	399
English muffin with butter	170	2	<1	5	45	9
hash brown potatoes	130	3	<1	7	60	9
hotcakes with butter and syrup	410	3	3	9	80	21
McMuffin, egg	290	4	1	11	100	226
sausage	370	8	2	22	200	64
sausage with egg	440	10	3	27	240	263
Sausage, pork, 1 serving	180	6	2	16	140	48
Wheaties, 1 box (⅘ oz)	90	<1	<1	<1	N.A.	0
Burgers						
Big Mac	560	10	2	32	290	103

*Less than 2% U.S. RDA

Sodium (mg)	Potassium (mg)	Protein (g)	Carbohy-drate (g)	Calcium (% U.S. RDA)	Iron (% U.S. RDA)	Vitamin A (% U.S. RDA)	Vitamin C (% U.S. RDA)
120	15	2	2	2	*	*	*
470	50	6	20	15	20	*	*
1110	800	18	82	35	20	4	2
1250	1030	25	85	35	20	4	2
1450	1170	31	89	35	25	4	2
330	120	2	9	6	4	15	*
230	N.A.	5	46	4	4	*	*
730	N.A.	5	32	8	8	*	*
1230	N.A.	18	33	20	15	10	*
1080	N.A.	13	32	8	15	*	*
1250	N.A.	20	33	10	20	6	*
210	N.A.	3	14	2	35	15	15
380	N.A.	6	53	2	10	2	10
290	N.A.	12	1	6	15	10	*
270	N.A.	5	27	15	10	2	*
330	N.A.	1	15	*	*	*	2
640	N.A.	8	74	10	15	4	*
740	N.A.	18	28	25	20	10	*
830	N.A.	17	27	25	15	4	*
980	N.A.	23	28	25	20	10	*
350	N.A.	8	0	*	*	*	*
220	N.A.	2	19	2	25	20	20
950	N.A.	25	43	25	25	8	2

~ MCDONALD'S/ PIZZA HUT†	Calories	Saturated fat (g)	Polyunsaturated fat (g)	Total fat (g)	Calories from fat	Cholesterol (mg)
cheeseburger	310	5	<1	14	130	53
hamburger	260	4	<1	10	90	37
McD.L.T.	580	12	9	37	330	109
McLean Deluxe	320	4	1	10	90	60
with cheese	370	5	1	14	130	75
Quarter Pounder	410	8	1	21	190	86
with cheese	520	11	2	29	260	118
Chicken						
McChicken Sandwich	490	5	12	29	260	43
McNuggets, 1 serving	290	4	2	16	140	65
Desserts						
cone, vanilla yogurt	100	<1	<1	<1	N.A.	3
Cookies, Chocolaty Chip	330	5	<1	16	140	4
McDonaldland	290	2	<1	9	80	0
milk shake, chocolate low-fat	320	<1	<1	2	18	10
strawberry low-fat	320	<1	<1	1	10	10
vanilla low-fat	290	<1	<1	1	10	10
pie, apple	260	5	<1	15	140	6
sundae, frozen yogurt						
hot caramel	270	2	<1	3	25	13
hot fudge	240	2	<1	3	25	6
strawberry	210	<1	0	1	10	5
Filet-O-Fish Sandwich	440	5	11	26	230	50
French fries, small	220	5	<1	12	110	9
medium	320	7	<1	17	150	12
large	400	9	<1	22	200	16
Salad, chef	230	6	<1	13	120	128
Salad, chunky chicken	140	<1	<1	3	25	78
Salad, garden	110	3	<1	7	60	83
Salad, side	60	2	<1	3	25	41
Hand-Tossed, cheese	520	14	N.A.	20	180	55

*Less than 2% U.S. RDA
†Except where noted, all values are based on 2 medium slices.

Sodium (mg)	Potassium (mg)	Protein (g)	Carbohy-drate (g)	Calcium (% U.S. RDA)	Iron (% U.S. RDA)	Vitamin A (% U.S. RDA)	Vitamin C (% U.S. RDA)
750	N.A.	15	31	20	15	8	4
500	N.A.	12	31	10	15	4	4
990	N.A.	26	36	25	25	15	15
670	290	22	35	15	20	10	10
890	310	24	35	20	20	15	10
660	N.A.	23	34	15	25	4	6
1150	N.A.	29	35	30	25	15	6
780	N.A.	19	40	15	20	2	4
520	N.A.	19	17	*	6	*	*
80	N.A.	4	22	10	*	2	*
280	N.A.	4	42	2	15	*	*
300	N.A.	4	47	*	15	*	*
240	N.A.	12	66	35	*	6	*
170	N.A.	11	67	35	*	6	*
170	N.A.	11	60	35	*	6	*
240	N.A.	2	30	*	4	*	20
180	N.A.	7	59	20	*	6	*
170	N.A.	7	51	25	4	4	*
95	N.A.	6	49	20	*	4	2
1030	N.A.	14	38	15	10	2	*
110	N.A.	3	26	*	4	*	15
150	N.A.	4	36	*	4	*	20
200	N.A.	6	46	*	6	*	25
490	N.A.	21	8	25	8	80	20
230	N.A.	23	5	4	6	70	20
160	N.A.	7	6	15	6	80	20
85	N.A.	4	3	8	4	45	10
1280	400	34	55	80	30	10	15

PIZZA HUT/ ROY ROGERS	Calories	Saturated fat (g)	Polyunsaturated fat (g)	Total fat (g)	Calories from fat	Cholesterol (mg)
pepperoni	500	13	N.A.	23	210	50
supreme	540	14	N.A.	26	230	55
super supreme	560	13	N.A.	25	230	54
Pan Pizza, cheese	490	9	N.A.	18	160	34
pepperoni	540	9	N.A.	22	200	42
supreme	590	14	N.A.	30	270	48
super supreme	560	12	N.A.	26	230	55
Personal Pan Pizza (whole pizza)						
pepperoni	680	13	N.A.	29	260	53
supreme	650	11	N.A.	29	260	49
Thin 'n Crispy, cheese	400	10	N.A.	17	150	33
pepperoni	410	11	N.A.	20	180	46
supreme	460	11	N.A.	22	200	42
super supreme	460	10	N.A.	21	190	56
Beef						
roast beef sandwich	320	N.A.	N.A.	10	90	55
with cheese	420	N.A.	N.A.	19	170	77
roast beef sandwich, large	360	N.A.	N.A.	12	110	73
with cheese	470	N.A.	N.A.	21	190	95
Biscuit	230	N.A.	N.A.	12	110	3
Breakfast items						
Breakfast Crescent Sandwich	400	N.A.	N.A.	27	240	148
with bacon	430	N.A.	N.A.	30	270	156
with ham	560	N.A.	N.A.	42	380	189
with sausage	450	N.A.	N.A.	29	260	168
crescent roll	290	N.A.	N.A.	18	160	3
danish, apple	250	N.A.	N.A.	12	110	15
cheese	250	N.A.	N.A.	12	110	11
cherry	270	N.A.	N.A.	14	130	11
egg and biscuit platter	390	N.A.	N.A.	27	240	284

*Less than 2% U.S. RDA

Sodium (mg)	Potassium (mg)	Protein (g)	Carbohy-drate (g)	Calcium (% U.S. RDA)	Iron (% U.S. RDA)	Vitamin A (% U.S. RDA)	Vitamin C (% U.S. RDA)
1270	420	28	50	45	30	10	10
1470	580	32	50	50	45	10	20
1650	520	33	54	45	40	10	20
940	340	30	57	70	30	10	10
1130	410	29	62	50	35	10	15
1360	580	32	53	50	30	10	15
1450	530	33	53	50	40	10	20
1340	400	37	76	70	30	10	15
1310	490	33	76	50	35	10	20
870	260	28	37	70	20	8	8
990	290	26	36	45	20	8	10
1330	540	28	41	45	35	10	15
1340	460	29	44	45	25	10	15
790	N.A.	27	29	8	25	2	*
1690	N.A.	33	30	35	25	8	*
1040	N.A.	34	30	8	25	2	*
1950	N.A.	40	30	35	25	8	*
580	N.A.	4	26	6	2	*	*
870	N.A.	13	25	15	8	10	*
1040	N.A.	15	26	15	10	10	*
1190	N.A.	20	25	15	10	10	*
1290	N.A.	20	26	15	10	10	*
550	N.A.	5	27	6	4	*	*
260	N.A.	5	32	10	6	2	*
260	N.A.	5	31	4	6	2	*
240	N.A.	4	32	4	6	4	*
730	N.A.	17	22	10	15	10	*

∼ ROY ROGERS

	Calories	Saturated fat (g)	Polyunsaturated fat (g)	Total fat (g)	Calories from fat	Cholesterol (mg)
with bacon	440	N.A.	N.A.	30	270	294
with ham	440	N.A.	N.A.	29	260	304
with sausage	550	N.A.	N.A.	41	370	325
Pancake platter (with syrup and butter)	450	N.A.	N.A.	15	140	53
with bacon	490	N.A.	N.A.	18	160	63
with ham	510	N.A.	N.A.	17	150	73
with sausage	610	N.A.	N.A.	30	270	94
Burgers						
bacon cheeseburger	580	N.A.	N.A.	39	350	103
cheeseburger	560	N.A.	N.A.	37	330	95
hamburger	460	N.A.	N.A.	28	250	73
RR Bar Burger	610	N.A.	N.A.	39	350	115
Chicken						
breast	320	N.A.	N.A.	19	170	324
breast and wing	470	N.A.	N.A.	29	260	376
leg	120	N.A.	N.A.	7	60	64
leg and thigh	400	N.A.	N.A.	26	230	153
thigh	280	N.A.	N.A.	20	180	89
wing	140	N.A.	N.A.	10	90	52
Cole slaw	110	N.A.	N.A.	7	60	3
Desserts						
brownie	260	N.A.	N.A.	11	100	10
milk shake, chocolate	360	N.A.	N.A.	10	90	37
strawberry	320	N.A.	N.A.	10	90	37
vanilla	310	N.A.	N.A.	11	100	40
strawberry shortcake	450	N.A.	N.A.	19	170	28
sundae, caramel	290	N.A.	N.A.	9	80	23
hot fudge	340	N.A.	N.A.	13	120	23
strawberry	220	N.A.	N.A.	7	60	23
French fries, regular serving	270	N.A.	N.A.	14	130	42
large	360	N.A.	N.A.	18	160	56

*Less than 2% U.S. RDA

Sodium (mg)	Potassium (mg)	Protein (g)	Carbohy-drate (g)	Calcium (% U.S. RDA)	Iron (% U.S. RDA)	Vitamin A (% U.S. RDA)	Vitamin C (% U.S. RDA)
960	N.A.	20	22	10	10	10	*
1160	N.A.	24	23	10	15	10	*
1060	N.A.	24	22	15	15	10	*
840	N.A.	8	72	10	10	20	*
1070	N.A.	10	72	10	10	20	*
1260	N.A.	14	72	10	15	20	*
1170	N.A.	14	72	10	15	20	*
1540	N.A.	32	25	35	25	8	*
1400	N.A.	30	27	35	20	8	*
500	N.A.	24	27	10	20	*	*
1830	N.A.	36	28	35	20	10	*
600	N.A.	32	7	4	6	*	*
870	N.A.	42	11	6	8	2	*
160	N.A.	12	2	*	2	*	*
670	N.A.	32	9	2	8	*	*
500	N.A.	20	7	*	6	*	*
270	N.A.	10	3	*	2	*	*
260	N.A.	1	11	4	*	8	140
150	N.A.	3	37	2	15	*	*
290	N.A.	8	61	30	2	8	*
260	N.A.	8	49	30	2	8	2
280	N.A.	8	45	30	2	10	*
670	N.A.	10	59	25	4	8	2
190	N.A.	7	52	20	2	8	*
190	N.A.	7	53	25	6	10	*
100	N.A.	6	33	20	2	8	2
170	N.A.	4	32	*	4	*	15
220	N.A.	5	43	2	4	*	20

～ ROY ROGERS/ SALAD BAR	Calories	Saturated fat (g)	Polyunsaturated fat (g)	Total fat (g)	Calories from fat	Cholesterol (mg)
Macaroni salad, 3½ oz	190	N.A.	N.A.	11	100	3
Potatoes						
hot topped potato, plain	210	N.A.	N.A.	<1	N.A.	0
with bacon and cheese	400	N.A.	N.A.	22	200	34
with broccoli and cheese	380	N.A.	N.A.	18	160	18
with oleo	270	N.A.	N.A.	7	60	0
with sour cream and chives	410	N.A.	N.A.	21	190	31
with taco beef and cheese	460	N.A.	N.A.	22	200	37
potato salad, 3½ oz	110	N.A.	N.A.	6	50	3
Alfalfa sprouts, 1 cup	8	0	0	0	N.A.	0
Applesauce, chunky, 2 tbsp	20	N.A.	N.A.	<1	N.A.	0
Bacon bits, 1 tbsp	40	5	2	14	130	10
Bananas, 1 oz—4 or 5 slices	25	N.A.	N.A.	<1	N.A.	0
Breadsticks, 2	30	<1	<1	1	10	0
Broccoli, ½ cup	12	0	0	0	N.A.	0
Cantaloupe, 2 pieces	20	0	0	0	N.A.	0
Carrots, ¼ cup	12	0	0	0	N.A.	0
Cauliflower, ½ cup	14	0	0	0	N.A.	0
Cheddar chips, ¼ cup	160	N.A.	N.A.	12	110	5
Cheese, shredded imitation, ¼ cup	90	4	0	6	50	<1
Chicken salad, ¼ cup	120	2	3	8	70	<1
Chives, 1 tbsp	8	N.A.	N.A.	<1	N.A.	0
Chow mein noodles, ⅓ cup	70	<1	2	4	35	0
Cole slaw, ¼ cup	70	<1	4	5	45	5
Cottage cheese, ½ cup	110	3	<1	4	35	15
Croutons, 1 tbsp	60	N.A.	N.A.	3	25	N.A.
Cucumbers, 4 slices	2	N.A.	N.A.	0	N.A.	0
Eggs, hard cooked, 1 tbsp	30	<1	<1	2	18	90
Garbanzo beans, 2 tbsp	45	<1	<1	1	10	0
Green peas, ⅓ cup	20	0	0	0	N.A.	0

*Less than 2% U.S. RDA

Sodium (mg)	Potassium (mg)	Protein (g)	Carbohy-drate (g)	Calcium (% U.S. RDA)	Iron (% U.S. RDA)	Vitamin A (% U.S. RDA)	Vitamin C (% U.S. RDA)
600	N.A.	3	19	*	2	*	*
65	N.A.	6	48	2	8	*	45
780	N.A.	17	33	15	10	4	8
520	N.A.	14	40	20	15	4	15
160	N.A.	6	48	2	8	6	60
140	N.A.	7	48	10	15	10	25
730	N.A.	22	45	15	20	4	20
700	N.A.	2	11	*	*	4	2
0	15	1	1	*	*	*	4
0	15	<1	6	*	*	*	*
350	45	5	<1	*	*	*	2
0	110	<1	7	*	*	*	4
30	15	1	5	2	2	*	*
10	140	1	2	2	2	6	70
5	180	<1	5	*	*	20	30
10	90	<1	2	*	*	80	4
10	200	1	3	2	2	*	70
450	50	3	12	6	2	*	*
125	0	6	1	20	*	4	*
220	60	7	4	*	2	*	4
0	90	<1	2	2	4	20	35
60	15	1	8	*	4	*	*
130	90	<1	8	2	*	4	25
430	90	13	3	6	*	6	*
160	30	2	8	*	4	*	*
0	20	<1	<1	*	*	*	*
25	25	3	<1	*	*	4	*
5	85	3	8	*	6	*	*
30	40	1	4	*	2	4	8

~ SALAD BAR

	Calories	Saturated fat (g)	Polyunsat-urated fat (g)	Total fat (g)	Calories from fat	Choles-terol (mg)
Green peppers, ¼ cup	10	0	0	0	N.A.	0
Honeydew melon, 2 pieces	20	0	0	0	N.A.	0
Jalapeño peppers, 1 tbsp	2	0	0	0	N.A.	0
Ketchup, 1 tbsp	18	0	0	0	N.A.	0
Lettuce, iceberg, 1 cup	8	0	0	0	N.A.	0
romaine, 1 cup	10	0	0	0	N.A.	0
Mayonnaise, 2 tbsp	190	4	14	21	190	16
Mushrooms, ¼ cup	4	0	0	0	N.A.	0
Mustard, ½ tsp	2	0	0	0	N.A.	0
Olives, black, 7 medium	35	<1	<1	3	25	0
Onions, red, 3 rings	2	0	0	0	N.A.	0
Oranges, ¼ cup	25	0	0	0	N.A.	0
Parmesan cheese, 1 tbsp	25	1	<1	2	18	4
imitation, 1 tbsp	14	N.A.	N.A.	<1	N.A.	<1
Pasta salad, ¼ cup	35	N.A.	N.A.	<1	N.A.	0
Peaches, ¼ cup	30	0	0	0	N.A.	0
Pepperoni, 5 slices	140	5	1	12	110	35
Pineapple chunks, ½ cup	60	0	0	0	N.A.	0
Potato salad, ¼ cup	130	<1	4	11	100	10
Pudding, butterscotch, ¼ cup	90	N.A.	N.A.	4	35	<1
chocolate, ¼ cup	90	N.A.	N.A.	4	35	<1
Red pepper, crushed, 1 tsp	8	N.A.	N.A.	<1	N.A.	0
Salad dressings, all 1 tbsp						
bacon and tomato, reduced-calorie	45	<1	3	4	35	<1
blue cheese	90	2	6	10	90	10
celery seed	70	<1	4	6	50	5
French	60	<1	4	6	50	0
French, sweet red	70	<1	4	6	50	0
hidden valley ranch	50	1	4	6	50	5
Italian caesar	80	1	5	9	80	5
Italian, golden	45	<1	2	4	35	0

*Less than 2% U.S. RDA

Sodium (mg)	Potassium (mg)	Protein (g)	Carbohy-drate (g)	Calcium (% U.S. RDA)	Iron (% U.S. RDA)	Vitamin A (% U.S. RDA)	Vitamin C (% U.S. RDA)
0	65	<1	2	*	*	2	60
5	160	<1	5	*	*	*	25
190	10	<1	<1	*	*	*	*
180	N.A.	0	4	*	*	6	8
5	85	<1	1	*	2	2	4
5	160	1	1	2	4	15	20
140	N.A.	0	2	*	*	*	*
0	65	<1	<1	*	*	*	*
35	N.A.	0	0	*	*	*	*
250	5	<1	2	2	4	*	*
0	15	<1	<1	*	*	*	*
0	100	<1	7	2	*	*	50
95	5	2	<1	8	*	*	*
75	15	2	<1	8	*	4	*
120	N.A.	2	6	*	2	*	*
5	55	<1	8	*	*	2	2
440	55	5	2	*	2	*	*
0	120	<1	16	*	2	*	15
90	135	<1	6	*	2	*	10
85	N.A.	1	11	6	2	*	*
70	N.A.	<1	12	15	2	*	*
0	0	<1	1	*	*	15	*
190	15	<1	3	*	*	*	*
110	10	<1	<1	*	*	*	*
65	10	<1	3	*	*	*	*
180	20	<1	4	*	*	*	*
125	15	<1	5	*	*	*	*
95	15	<1	<1	*	*	*	*
140	5	<1	<1	*	*	*	*
250	10	<1	3	*	*	*	*

~ SALAD BAR/ TACO BELL†	Calories	Saturated fat (g)	Polyunsat-urated fat (g)	Total fat (g)	Calories from fat	Choles-terol (mg)
Italian, reduced-calorie	25	<1	2	2	18	0
salad oil	130	2	5	14	130	0
Thousand Island	70	1	4	7	60	5
wine vinegar	2	0	0	0	N.A.	0
Sauces, dipping, all 2 tbsp						
barbeque	50	N.A.	N.A.	<1	N.A.	0
honey	90	N.A.	N.A.	<1	N.A.	0
sweet mustard	50	<1	<1	1	10	0
sweet and sour	45	N.A.	N.A.	<1	N.A.	0
tartar	170	3	11	18	160	16
Seafood salad, ¼ cup	110	<1	4	7	60	<1
Sour cream topping, 2 tbsp	60	5	<1	5	45	0
Strawberries, ⅓ cup	18	0	0	0	N.A.	0
Sunflower seeds and raisins, 3 tbsp	140	7	1	10	90	0
Three bean salad, ¼ cup	60	N.A.	N.A.	<1	N.A.	N.A.
Tomatoes, ¼ cup	6	0	0	0	N.A.	0
Tuna salad, ¼ cup	100	<1	3	6	50	<1
Turkey ham, ¼ cup	35	<1	<1	1	10	15
Watermelon, 2 pieces	18	0	0	0	N.A.	0
Burrito, bean, with green sauce	350	3	2	10	90	9
with red sauce	360	3	2	10	90	9
Burrito, beef, with green sauce	400	7	2	17	150	57
with red sauce	400	7	2	17	150	57
Burrito Supreme, with green sauce	410	8	2	18	160	33
with red sauce	410	8	2	18	160	33
Cinnamon Crispas	260	4	<1	15	140	<1
Double Beef Burrito Supreme, with green sauce	450	10	2	22	200	57
with red sauce	460	10	2	22	200	57
Enchirito, with green sauce	370	9	2	20	180	54

*Less than 2% U.S. RDA
†All values base on 1 item or 1 serving unless otherwise noted.

Sodium (mg)	Potassium (mg)	Protein (g)	Carbohy-drate (g)	Calcium (% U.S. RDA)	Iron (% U.S. RDA)	Vitamin A (% U.S. RDA)	Vitamin C (% U.S. RDA)
190	10	<1	2	*	*	*	*
0	0	0	0	*	*	*	*
110	15	<1	2	*	*	*	*
5	10	<1	<1	*	*	*	*
100	95	<1	11	*	4	6	*
10	0	<1	24	*	*	*	*
140	30	<1	9	*	*	*	*
55	40	<1	11	*	2	*	*
300	N.A.	0	3	*	*	*	*
460	40	4	7	20	2	*	2
30	45	<1	2	*	*	*	*
0	95	<1	4	*	*	*	50
5	240	5	6	2	10	*	*
15	55	1	13	*	2	4	*
5	65	<1	1	*	*	2	10
290	90	8	4	*	2	*	4
280	80	5	<1	*	4	*	*
0	65	<1	4	*	*	2	10
760	390	13	53	15	20	4	90
890	430	13	54	15	20	8	90
930	280	22	38	10	20	6	*
1050	310	23	39	10	20	10	2
800	400	18	45	15	20	15	40
920	430	18	47	15	20	20	45
130	35	3	28	4	8	*	*
930	400	23	40	15	20	15	15
1050	430	24	42	15	20	20	15
990	350	20	28	25	15	15	45

~ TACO BELL/ WENDY'S	Calories	Saturated fat (g)	Polyunsat- urated fat (g)	Total fat (g)	Calories from fat	Choles- terol (mg)
with red sauce	380	9	2	20	180	54
Guacamole (¾ oz)	35	<1	<1	2	18	0
Jalapeño peppers (3½ oz)	20	<1	0	<1	N.A.	0
Mexican pizza	580	11	10	37	330	52
Meximelt (3¾ oz)	270	8	2	15	140	38
Nachos	350	6	2	19	170	9
Nachos Bellegrande	650	12	3	35	320	36
Pico de Gallo (1 oz)	8	0	<1	<1	N.A.	<1
Pintos and cheese, with green sauce	180	4	<1	8	70	16
with red sauce	190	4	<1	9	80	16
Ranch dressing (2½ oz)	240	5	14	25	230	36
Salsa (⅓ oz)	18	0	0	<1	N.A.	0
Sour cream (¾ oz)	45	3	N.A.	4	35	N.A.
Taco, regular	180	5	<1	11	100	32
light	410	12	5	29	260	56
soft	230	5	1	12	110	32
soft supreme	280	8	1	16	140	32
super combo	290	7	1	16	140	40
Taco Bellegrande	360	11	1	23	210	56
Taco, chicken	210	4	2	10	90	43
Taco salad, no shell	500	14	2	31	280	80
with salsa, no shell	520	14	2	31	280	80
with salsa and shell	940	19	12	61	550	80
Taco sauce, 1 packet	4	0	0	<1	N.A.	0
Taco, steak	220	5	1	11	100	14
Tostada, with green sauce	240	4	<1	11	100	16
with red sauce	240	4	<1	11	100	16
Chicken, Crispy Nuggets, 6 pc	280	5	4	20	180	50
Chili, regular	220	3	<1	7	60	45
large	330	4	<1	11	100	68

*Less than 2% U.S. RDA

Sodium (mg)	Potassium (mg)	Protein (g)	Carbohy-drate (g)	Calcium (% U.S. RDA)	Iron (% U.S. RDA)	Vitamin A (% U.S. RDA)	Vitamin C (% U.S. RDA)
1240	420	20	31	25	15	20	45
115	110	<1	3	*	*	2	6
1370	110	1	4	4	*	6	4
1030	410	21	40	25	20	20	50
690	115	13	19	25	10	15	2
400	160	8	38	20	6	10	4
1000	670	22	61	30	20	25	100
90	0	<1	1	*	*	10	2
520	350	9	18	15	8	6	90
640	380	9	19	15	8	8	90
570	45	2	2	2	2	4	*
380	380	1	4	4	4	20	4
N.A.	30	<1	<1	2	*	4	*
280	160	10	11	8	6	6	2
590	320	19	18	15	15	15	8
520	180	12	18	10	15	4	2
520	230	13	19	15	15	8	4
460	290	14	21	15	10	15	25
470	330	18	18	20	10	15	10
550	190	13	18	10	10	6	4
1060	990	30	26	35	25	40	120
1430	1150	31	30	35	30	60	130
1660	1210	36	63	40	40	60	130
105	15	<1	<1	*	*	4	*
420	190	14	18	10	15	4	2
470	370	9	25	15	8	10	70
600	400	10	27	20	8	15	80
600	200	14	12	4	4	*	*
750	500	21	23	8	35	15	15
1130	740	32	35	10	50	25	25

✺ WENDY'S

	Calories	Saturated fat (g)	Polyunsat-urated fat (g)	Total fat (g)	Calories from fat	Choles-terol (mg)
cheddar cheese, shredded (¼ cup)	110	6	<1	10	90	30
sour cream (2 tbsp)	60	4	<1	6	35	10
Chocolate chip cookie	280	4	3	13	120	15
French fries, small	240	3	<1	12	110	0
large	310	3	1	16	140	0
biggie	450	5	1	22	200	0
Frosty Dairy Dessert, small	400	5	<1	14	130	50
medium	520	6	<1	18	160	65
large	680	8	<1	24	220	85
Potatoes, hot stuffed, plain	270	N.A.	N.A.	<1	N.A.	0
with bacon and cheese	520	5	8	18	160	20
with broccoli and cheese	400	3	7	16	140	<1
with cheese	420	4	7	15	140	10
with chili and cheese	500	4	3	18	160	25
with sour cream and chives	500	9	7	23	210	25
Salads, prepared						
chef salad	180	N.A.	N.A.	9	80	120
garden salad	100	N.A.	N.A.	5	45	0
taco salad	660	N.A.	N.A.	37	330	35
Sandwich makings (assembled to your specification)						
bacon slice	30	1	<1	3	25	5
cheese slice (American)	70	4	1	6	50	15
chicken fillet, grilled	100	<1	<1	3	25	55
chicken breast fillet (breaded and fried)	220	2	2	10	90	55
hamburger patty (¼ lb)	180	5	<1	12	110	65
kaiser bun	200	1	1	3	25	10
white bun	160	1	1	3	25	<1
Sandwiches						
Big Classic	570	6	1	33	300	90
chicken (breaded and fried)	430	3	3	19	170	60

*Less than 2% U.S. RDA

Sodium (mg)	Potassium (mg)	Protein (g)	Carbohy-drate (g)	Calcium (% U.S. RDA)	Iron (% U.S. RDA)	Vitamin A (% U.S. RDA)	Vitamin C (% U.S. RDA)
180	30	7	1	20	*	10	*
15	40	1	1	4	*	6	*
260	70	3	40	2	8	2	*
150	510	3	33	*	4	*	10
190	660	4	43	*	6	*	15
270	950	6	62	*	8	*	20
220	590	8	59	30	6	10	*
290	760	10	77	40	8	15	N.A.
370	990	14	100	50	10	15	N.A.
20	1050	6	63	2	20	*	50
1460	1350	20	70	8	25	10	60
460	1530	8	58	10	15	15	60
310	1080	8	66	6	20	10	50
630	1270	15	71	8	30	15	60
135	1190	8	67	10	20	50	80
140	590	15	10	25	15	110	110
110	560	7	9	20	10	110	110
1110	1330	40	46	80	35	80	80
100	30	2	<1	*	*	*	4
260	30	4	<1	10	*	6	*
330	210	18	<1	*	6	*	*
400	270	21	11	*	70	*	*
210	210	19	<1	*	20	*	*
350	70	6	37	10	10	*	*
290	60	5	30	10	10	*	*
1090	530	27	47	15	35	10	20
730	390	26	41	10	80	2	8

∾ WENDY'S

	Calories	Saturated fat (g)	Polyunsaturated fat (g)	Total fat (g)	Calories from fat	Cholesterol (mg)
chicken (grilled)	340	3	6	13	120	60
chicken club	510	5	4	25	230	70
fish fillet	460	5	9	25	230	55
junior hamburger (2 oz beef)	260	3	1	9	80	34
junior cheeseburger (2 oz beef)	310	3	1	13	120	34
junior bacon cheeseburger (2 oz beef)	430	6	2	25	230	50
junior Swiss deluxe (2 oz beef)	360	3	1	18	160	40
kids' meal hamburger (2 oz beef)	260	3	1	9	80	35
kids' meal cheeseburger (2 oz beef)	300	3	1	13	120	35
single (4 oz beef), plain	340	6	1	15	140	65
with everything	420	6	1	21	190	70

*Less than 2% U.S. RDA

Sodium (mg)	Potassium (mg)	Protein (g)	Carbohy-drate (g)	Calcium (% U.S. RDA)	Iron (% U.S. RDA)	Vitamin A (% U.S. RDA)	Vitamin C (% U.S. RDA)
820	340	24	36	10	20	2	8
930	450	30	42	10	80	2	15
780	320	18	42	10	15	2	2
570	220	15	33	10	20	2	4
770	220	18	33	10	20	2	4
840	290	22	32	10	20	2	15
770	290	18	34	20	20	4	10
570	210	15	32	10	20	2	2
770	210	18	33	10	20	2	2
500	280	24	30	10	30	*	*
890	430	25	35	10	30	5	15

~FATS

~OILS

~MARGARINES

~& SALAD

DRESSINGS

~ Fats are not a source of fiber. Some prepared dressings contain sugar, but listings for amounts are not readily available.

~ FATS, OILS, MARGARINES & SALAD DRESSINGS	Calories	Saturated fat (g)	Polyunsat- urated fat (g)	Total fat (g)	Calories from fat	Choles- terol (mg)
Beef tallow, 1 tbsp	120	6	<1	13	120	14
Butter, regular, 1 pat (1 tsp) (unsalted contains 0 mg sodium)	35	3	<1	4	35	35
1 stick (8 tbsp) (unsalted contains 12 mg sodium)	810	57	3	92	810	248
Butter, whipped, 1 pat (1 tsp)	25	2	<1	3	25	8
1 stick (8 tbsp)	540	38	2	60	540	165
Chicken fat, 1 tbsp	120	4	3	13	120	11
Creamer, non-dairy, liquid frozen, ½ oz (1 tbsp)	20	<1	0	2	18	0
powdered, 1 tsp	12	<1	0	<1	N.A.	0
refrigerated Coffee Mate (Carnation), 1 tbsp	16	<1	<1	1	10	0
Cream, half and half, 1 tbsp	20	1	<1	2	18	6
light table cream, 1 tbsp	30	2	<1	3	25	10
light whipping cream, 1 cup (2 cups whipped)	700	46	2	74	670	270
heavy whipping cream, 1 cup (2 cups whipped)	820	55	3	88	790	326
Lard (pork fat), 1 tbsp	120	5	1	13	120	12
Margarines						
regular, hard stick or soft tub, 1 tsp (unsalted has 0 mg sodium)	35	<1	2	4	35	0
spread or "light" (60% fat), 1 tsp	25	<1	<1	3	25	0
diet or "extra light" (40% fat), 1 tsp	18	<1	<1	2	18	0
liquid, 1 tsp	35	<1	2	4	35	0
butter blends, 1 tsp (unsalted has 0 mg sodium)	35	1	1	4	35	5
light, 1 tsp	20	1	1	2	18	3
Mayonnaise, regular, 1 tbsp	100	2	6	11	100	8
fat free, Kraft Free, 1 tbsp	12	0	0	0	0	0

*Less than 2% U.S. RDA

Sodium (mg)	Potassium (mg)	Protein (g)	Carbohy-drate (g)	Calcium (% U.S. RDA)	Iron (% U.S. RDA)	Vitamin A (% U.S. RDA)	Vitamin C (% U.S. RDA)
0	0	0	0	N.A.	N.A.	N.A.	N.A.
40	0	<1	0	*	*	4	*
940	30	1	<1	2	*	70	*
30	0	0	0	*	*	2	*
630	20	<1	N.A.	2	*	45	*
N.A.	N.A.	0	0	N.A.	N.A.	N.A.	N.A.
10	30	<1	2	*	*	*	*
0	15	<1	1	*	*	*	*
5	20	0	2	*	*	*	*
5	20	<1	<1	2	*	*	*
5	20	<1	<1	*	*	2	*
80	230	5	7	15	*	50	2
90	180	5	7	15	*	70	2
0	0	0	0	N.A.	N.A.	N.A.	N.A.
50	0	0	0	*	N.A.	4	*
50	0	0	0	*	N.A.	4	*
45	0	0	0	*	N.A.	4	*
35	45	<1	0	*	N.A.	4	*
35	N.A.	0	0	*	*	4	*
30	N.A.	0	0	*	*	4	*
80	5	<1	<1	*	*	*	N.A.
190	N.A.	0	3	*	*	*	*

FATS, OILS, MARGARINES & SALAD DRESSINGS	Calories	Saturated fat (g)	Polyunsat-urated fat (g)	Total fat (g)	Calories from fat	Choles-terol (mg)
light reduced calorie, Hellmann's, 1 tbsp (cholesterol-free has 0 mg cholesterol, 80 mg sodium)	50	1	2	5	45	5
Nuts (see Legumes & Seeds)						
Oil, all 1 tbsp						
canola (Wesson)	120	4	1	13	120	0
coconut	120	12	<1	13	120	0
corn	120	2	8	13	120	0
cottonseed	120	4	7	13	120	0
olive	120	2	1	13	120	0
palm	120	7	1	13	120	0
palm kernel	120	11	<1	13	120	0
peanut	120	2	4	13	120	0
safflower	120	1	10	13	120	0
sesame	120	2	6	13	120	0
soybean	120	2	8	13	120	0
sunflower	120	1	9	13	120	0
Olives (see Condiments, Sauces, Gravies & Seasonings)						
Salad dressing, bottled						
regular dressing, 1 tbsp, all varieties	80	1	4	7	60	3
low-calorie, 1 tbsp, all varieties	20	<1	<1	2	18	1
no-fat, Hidden Valley Take Heart, 1 tbsp, all varieties (ranch contains 1 gram fat)	18	0	0	0	0	0
Salad dressing, mayonnaise type, 1 tbsp	60	<1	3	5	45	4
Kraft Miracle Whip Free, 1 tbsp, no-fat	20	0	0	0	0	0
Salad dressing mix						

*Less than 2% U.S. RDA

Sodium (mg)	Potassium (mg)	Protein (g)	Carbohy-drate (g)	Calcium (% U.S. RDA)	Iron (% U.S. RDA)	Vitamin A (% U.S. RDA)	Vitamin C (% U.S. RDA)
115	N.A.	0	1	*	*	*	*
0	0	0	0	*	*	*	*
N.A.	N.A.	0	0	N.A.	N.A.	N.A.	N.A.
N.A.	N.A.	0	0	N.A.	N.A.	N.A.	N.A.
N.A.	N.A.	0	0	N.A.	N.A.	N.A.	N.A.
0	N.A.	0	0	*	*	N.A.	N.A.
N.A.	N.A.	0	0	N.A.	N.A.	N.A.	N.A.
N.A.	N.A.	0	0	N.A.	N.A.	N.A.	N.A.
0	0	0	0	*	*	N.A.	N.A.
N.A.	N.A.	0	0	N.A.	N.A.	N.A.	N.A.
N.A.	N.A.	0	0	N.A.	N.A.	N.A.	N.A.
0	N.A.	0	0	*	*	N.A.	N.A.
N.A.	N.A.	0	0	N.A.	N.A.	N.A.	N.A.
150	15	<1	2	*	*	*	*
135	N.A.	<1	3	*	*	N.A.	N.A.
135	N.A.	0	3	*	*	*	*
105	0	<1	4	*	*	*	N.A.
210	N.A.	0	5	*	*	*	*

~ FATS, OILS, MARGARINES & SALAD DRESSINGS	Calories	Saturated fat (g)	Polyunsat-urated fat (g)	Total fat (g)	Calories from fat	Choles-terol (mg)
Good Seasons (General Foods), 1 tbsp	70	N.A.	N.A.	7	60	3
lite, 1 tbsp, all flavors	30	N.A.	N.A.	3	25	3
Hidden Valley, 1 tbsp, buttermilk recipe	60	N.A.	N.A.	3	25	4
made with mayon-naise-type salad dressing	35	N.A.	N.A.	3	25	3
Shortening, hydrogenated vegetable (Crisco), 1 tbsp	110	3	3	12	110	0
lard and vegetable oil mixture, 1 tbsp	120	5	1	13	120	N.A.
Sour cream, cultured, 1 tbsp	25	2	<1	3	25	5
imitation, 1 oz (2⅓ tbsp)	60	5	<1	6	50	0
non-butterfat sour dressing, 1 tbsp	20	2	<1	2	18	1
Topping, whipped real cream, 1 tbsp	8	<1	<1	<1	N.A.	2
Topping, whipped frozen, 1 tbsp	14	<1	<1	1	10	0
1 cup	240	16	<1	19	170	0
powdered non-dairy topping, 1 tbsp prepared	8	<1	<1	<1	N.A.	0
1 cup	150	9	<1	10	90	8
pressurized, 1 tbsp	12	<1	<1	<1	N.A.	0

*Less than 2% U.S. RDA

Sodium (mg)	Potassium (mg)	Protein (g)	Carbohy-drate (g)	Calcium (% U.S. RDA)	Iron (% U.S. RDA)	Vitamin A (% U.S. RDA)	Vitamin C (% U.S. RDA)
150	15	1	1	*	*	*	*
150	15	1	2	*	*	*	*
110	N.A.	0	1	N.A.	N.A.	N.A.	N.A.
120	N.A.	0	2	N.A.	N.A.	N.A.	N.A.
0	N.A.	0	0	*	*	*	*
N.A.	N.A.	0	0	N.A.	N.A.	N.A.	N.A.
5	15	<1	<1	*	*	2	*
30	45	<1	2	*	N.A.	*	*
5	20	<1	<1	*	*	*	*
0	0	<1	<1	*	*	*	*
0	0	<1	<1	*	*	*	*
20	15	1	17	*	*	15	*
0	5	<1	<1	*	*	*	*
55	120	3	13	8	*	6	*
0	0	<1	<1	*	*	*	*

~FRUITS

~& FRUIT JUICES

~ *Values for fiber and sugar content are listed where available.*

~ FRUITS & FRUIT JUICES	Calories	Saturated fat (g)	Polyunsaturated fat (g)	Total fat (g)	Calories from fat	Cholesterol (mg)
Apple, fresh, raw with skin, 2¾" (⅓ lb)	80	N.A.	N.A.	<1	N.A.	0
boiled without skin, ½ cup	45	N.A.	N.A.	<1	N.A.	0
canned sweetened, sliced, ½ cup	70	N.A.	N.A.	<1	N.A.	0
chips, Weight Watchers, 1 bag (¾ oz)	70	N.A.	N.A.	0	N.A.	N.A.
dehydrated, ½ cup (1 oz)	100	N.A.	N.A.	<1	N.A.	0
dried, 10 rings (2¼ oz)	160	N.A.	N.A.	<1	N.A.	0
glazed in raspberry sauce, Budget Gourmet, frozen side dish	110	N.A.	N.A.	3	25	10
Apple fritters, Mrs. Paul's, 2 fritters	270	N.A.	N.A.	13	120	N.A.
Apple juice, canned or bottled, 1 cup	120	N.A.	N.A.	<1	N.A.	0
frozen concentrate, diluted with 3 parts water, 1 cup	110	N.A.	N.A.	<1	N.A.	0
Applesauce, canned, unsweetened, ½ cup	50	N.A.	N.A.	<1	N.A.	0
sweetened, ½ cup	100	N.A.	N.A.	<1	N.A.	0
Apricots, fresh, 1 cup halves (8 halves)	70	N.A.	N.A.	<1	N.A.	0
canned water pack, 1 cup	70	N.A.	N.A.	<1	N.A.	0
in light syrup, 1 cup	160	N.A.	N.A.	<1	N.A.	0
in heavy syrup, 1 cup	210	N.A.	N.A.	<1	N.A.	0
dried, 1 cup	310	N.A.	N.A.	<1	N.A.	0
Apricot nectar, canned, 1 cup	140	N.A.	N.A.	<1	N.A.	0
Avocado, 1 (9¼ oz)	320	5	4	31	280	0
puree, 1 cup	370	6	4	35	320	0
Banana, fresh, 8¾" long	110	N.A.	N.A.	<1	N.A.	0
1 cup mashed	210	N.A.	N.A.	1	10	0
dehydrated, 1 cup	350	N.A.	N.A.	2	18	0
Blackberries, fresh, ½ cup raw	35	N.A.	N.A.	<1	N.A.	0

*Less than 2% U.S. RDA

Sodium (mg)	Potassium (mg)	Protein (g)	Carbohydrate (g)	Dietary fiber (g)	Sugars (g)	Calcium (% U.S. RDA)	Iron (% U.S. RDA)	Vitamin A (% U.S. RDA)	Vitamin C (% U.S. RDA)
0	160	<1	21	4.2	18	*	*	*	15
0	75	<1	12	2.1	N.A.	*	*	*	*
0	70	<1	17	2.2	N.A.	*	*	*	*
200	N.A.	0	19	N.A.	N.A.	*	*	*	6
40	200	<1	28	N.A.	N.A.	*	4	*	*
55	290	<1	42	N.A.	N.A.	*	6	*	4
210	N.A.	0	22	N.A.	N.A.	4	4	*	200
610	N.A.	3	36	N.A.	N.A.	2	8	*	6
5	300	<1	29	N.A.	27	*	6	*	4
15	300	<1	28	N.A.	N.A.	*	4	N.A.	2
0	90	<1	14	2	N.A.	*	*	*	2
0	80	<1	25	1.8	21	*	4	*	4
0	460	2	17	2	3	2	6	80	25
5	470	2	16	N.A.	N.A.	2	6	6	15
10	350	1	42	N.A.	N.A.	2	6	70	10
10	360	1	55	N.A.	N.A.	2	6	60	15
15	1790	5	80	9.5	N.A.	6	40	190	6
10	290	1	36	N.A.	N.A.	2	5	70	2
20	1200	4	15	8.8	N.A.	2	15	25	25
25	1380	5	17	N.A.	N.A.	2	15	30	30
0	450	1	27	1.6	18	*	2	2	20
0	890	2	53	3.2	N.A.	*	4	4	35
0	1490	4	88	N.A.	N.A.	2	8	6	10
0	140	1	9	3.2	N.A.	2	2	2	25

∿ FRUITS & FRUIT JUICES	Calories	Saturated fat (g)	Polyunsaturated fat (g)	Total fat (g)	Calories from fat	Cholesterol (mg)
canned in heavy syrup, ½ cup	120	N.A.	N.A.	<1	N.A.	0
frozen, unsweetened, 1 cup	100	N.A.	N.A.	<1	N.A.	0
Blueberries, fresh, 1 cup raw	80	N.A.	N.A.	<1	N.A.	0
canned in heavy syrup, ½ cup	110	N.A.	N.A.	<1	N.A.	0
frozen, unsweetened, 1 cup	80	N.A.	N.A.	1	10	0
Cherries, sour, 1 cup fresh raw	50	N.A.	N.A.	<1	N.A.	0
canned water pack, ½ cup	45	N.A.	N.A.	<1	N.A.	0
in light syrup, ½ cup	90	N.A.	N.A.	<1	N.A.	0
in heavy syrup, ½ cup	120	N.A.	N.A.	<1	N.A.	0
frozen unsweetened, 1 cup	70	N.A.	N.A.	<1	N.A.	0
sweet, 10 fresh (2⅓ oz)	50	N.A.	N.A.	<1	N.A.	0
canned water pack, ½ cup	60	N.A.	N.A.	<1	N.A.	0
juice pack, ½ cup	70	N.A.	N.A.	<1	N.A.	0
in heavy syrup, ½ cup	110	N.A.	N.A.	<1	N.A.	0
frozen, sweetened, 1 cup	230	N.A.	N.A.	<1	N.A.	0
Cranberries, raw, 1 cup	45	N.A.	N.A.	<1	N.A.	0
Cranberry juice cocktail, bottled, 1 cup	140	0	0	0	0	0
frozen, prepared with water, 1 cup	130	0	0	0	0	0
low-calorie, with saccharin, 1 cup	45	0	0	0	0	0
Cranberry orange relish, canned, ½ cup	250	N.A.	N.A.	<1	N.A.	0
Cranberry sauce, canned, sweetened, ½ cup	210	N.A.	N.A.	<1	N.A.	0
Currants, black, ½ cup	35	N.A.	N.A.	<1	N.A.	0
red, white, ½ cup	30	N.A.	N.A.	<1	N.A.	0
Dates, natural and dry, 1 cup, chopped	490	N.A.	N.A.	<1	N.A.	0

*Less than 2% U.S. RDA

Sodium (mg)	Potassium (mg)	Protein (g)	Carbohy-drate (g)	Dietary fiber (g)	Sugars (g)	Calcium (% U.S. RDA)	Iron (% U.S. RDA)	Vitamin A (% U.S. RDA)	Vitamin C (% U.S. RDA)
0	125	2	30	N.A.	N.A.	2	6	6	6
0	210	2	24	N.A.	N.A.	4	8	4	8
10	130	1	20	4.4	11	*	*	2	30
0	50	1	28	N.A.	N.A.	*	2	2	2
0	85	1	19	5	N.A.	*	2	2	6
0	180	1	13	N.A.	9	2	2	25	15
10	120	1	11	1.8	N.A.	*	10	20	4
10	120	1	24	N.A.	N.A.	*	10	20	4
10	120	1	30	N.A.	N.A.	*	10	20	4
0	190	1	17	N.A.	N.A.	2	6	25	4
0	150	1	11	1	10	*	2	2	8
0	160	1	15	N.A.	N.A.	*	4	4	4
0	160	1	17	0.4	N.A.	*	4	4	6
0	190	1	27	N.A.	N.A.	*	4	4	8
0	510	3	58	N.A.	N.A.	4	6	10	4
0	65	<1	12	2.9	N.A.	*	*	*	20
5	45	0	36	N.A.	N.A.	*	2	*	150
10	35	0	34	N.A.	N.A.	*	2	*	40
10	50	0	11	N.A.	N.A.	2	*	N.A.	N.A.
45	55	<1	64	N.A.	N.A.	*	2	2	40
40	35	<1	54	N.A.	N.A.	*	2	*	4
0	180	<1	9	3	5	4	N.A.	2	170
0	150	<1	8	1.9	N.A.	2	4	*	40
5	1160	4	131	9.1	N.A.	6	15	2	*

~ FRUITS & FRUIT JUICES	Calories	Saturated fat (g)	Polyunsaturated fat (g)	Total fat (g)	Calories from fat	Cholesterol (mg)
10 fruits (3 oz)	230	N.A.	N.A.	<1	N.A.	0
Elderberries, 1 cup raw	110	N.A.	N.A.	<1	N.A.	0
Figs, fresh, 1 medium raw (1¾ oz)	35	N.A.	N.A.	<1	N.A.	0
canned water pack, 1 cup	130	N.A.	N.A.	<1	N.A.	0
in light syrup, 1 cup	170	N.A.	N.A.	<1	N.A.	0
in heavy syrup, 1 cup	230	N.A.	N.A.	<1	N.A.	0
dried, 10 (6½ oz)	480	<1	1	2	18	0
Fruit cocktail, canned, water pack, ½ cup	40	N.A.	N.A.	<1	N.A.	0
juice pack, ½ cup	60	N.A.	N.A.	<1	N.A.	0
in light syrup, ½ cup	70	N.A.	N.A.	<1	N.A.	0
in heavy syrup, ½ cup	90	N.A.	N.A.	<1	N.A.	0
Fruit snacks, Weight Watchers, 1 pouch (½ oz), all flavors	50	N.A.	N.A.	<1	N.A.	N.A.
Fruit spreads, Weight Watchers, 2 tsp, all flavors	16	0	0	0	0	N.A.
Grapefruit, fresh, ½ raw (3¾″ diameter)	40	N.A.	N.A.	<1	N.A.	0
canned water pack, ½ cup	45	N.A.	N.A.	<1	N.A.	0
juice pack, ½ cup	45	N.A.	N.A.	<1	N.A.	0
in light syrup, ½ cup	80	N.A.	N.A.	<1	N.A.	0
Grapefruit juice, fresh, 1 cup	100	N.A.	N.A.	<1	N.A.	0
canned unsweetened, 1 cup	90	N.A.	N.A.	<1	N.A.	0
sweetened, 1 cup	120	N.A.	N.A.	<1	N.A.	0
frozen concentrate, diluted with 3 parts water, 1 cup	100	N.A.	N.A.	<1	N.A.	0
Grapes, adherent skin (European type), 1 cup	110	N.A.	N.A.	1	10	0
slip skin (American type), 1 cup	60	N.A.	N.A.	<1	N.A.	0
Grape juice, canned or bottled, 1 cup	160	N.A.	N.A.	<1	N.A.	0

*Less than 2% U.S. RDA

Sodium (mg)	Potassium (mg)	Protein (g)	Carbohy-drate (g)	Dietary fiber (g)	Sugars (g)	Calcium (% U.S. RDA)	Iron (% U.S. RDA)	Vitamin A (% U.S. RDA)	Vitamin C (% U.S. RDA)
0	540	2	61	4.2	53	2	6	*	*
N.A.	410	1	27	N.A.	N.A.	6	15	15	90
0	115	<1	10	1.4	N.A.	2	*	*	2
0	260	1	35	N.A.	N.A.	6	4	2	4
0	260	1	45	N.A.	N.A.	6	4	2	4
0	260	1	59	N.A.	N.A.	6	4	2	4
20	1330	6	122	14	124	30	30	4	2
5	115	<1	10	N.A.	N.A.	*	2	6	4
0	120	<1	15	0.7	19	*	2	8	6
5	110	<1	19	N.A.	N.A.	*	2	6	4
5	110	<1	24	N.A.	N.A.	*	2	6	4
75	N.A.	<1	13	N.A.	N.A.	*	*	*	2
0	N.A.	0	4	N.A.	N.A.	*	*	*	*
0	170	<1	10	0.2	7	*	*	2	70
0	160	<1	11	N.A.	N.A.	2	4	*	45
10	210	1	11	0.2	N.A.	2	2	*	70
0	160	<1	20	N.A.	N.A.	2	4	*	45
0	400	1	23	N.A.	N.A.	2	4	N.A.	160
0	380	1	22	N.A.	N.A.	2	4	*	120
0	410	2	28	N.A.	19	2	6	*	110
0	340	1	24	N.A.	N.A.	2	2	*	140
0	300	1	28	2.7	N.A.	2	2	2	30
0	180	<1	16	N.A.	15	*	2	2	6
5	330	1	38	N.A.	N.A.	2	4	*	*

~ FRUITS & FRUIT JUICES	Calories	Saturated fat (g)	Polyunsat- urated fat (g)	Total fat (g)	Calories from fat	Choles- terol (mg)
frozen sweetened concentrate, diluted with 3 parts water, 1 cup	130	N.A.	N.A.	<1	N.A.	0
Guava, 1 fresh (4 oz)	45	N.A.	N.A.	<1	N.A.	0
Juice Bowl, Campbell's, 6 oz, all varieties	100	0	0	0	0	N.A.
Kiwi, 1 medium (3 oz)	45	N.A.	N.A.	<1	N.A.	0
Kumquat, 1 fresh (¾ oz)	12	N.A.	N.A.	<1	N.A.	0
Lemon, 1 medium (3¾ oz), with peel	20	N.A.	N.A.	<1	N.A.	0
edible portion	18	N.A.	N.A.	<1	N.A.	0
peel, 1 tbsp	0	0	0	0	0	0
Lemon juice, fresh, 1 tbsp	4	0	0	0	0	0
canned or bottled, 1 tbsp	4	0	0	0	0	0
Lime, 1 fresh (2¾ oz)	20	N.A.	N.A.	<1	N.A.	0
Lime juice, fresh, 1 tbsp	4	0	0	0	0	0
canned or bottled, 1 tbsp	4	0	0	0	0	0
Mango, 1 fresh (10½ oz)	140	N.A.	N.A.	<1	N.A.	0
Melon, all 1 cup pieces						
cantaloupe	60	N.A.	N.A.	<1	N.A.	0
casaba	45	N.A.	N.A.	<1	N.A.	0
honeydew	60	N.A.	N.A.	<1	N.A.	0
watermelon	50	N.A.	N.A.	<1	N.A.	0
Mixed fruit, canned in heavy syrup, ½ cup	90	N.A.	N.A.	<1	N.A.	0
dried, 11-oz pkg	710	<1	<1	1	10	0
frozen sweetened, 1 cup	250	N.A.	N.A.	<1	N.A.	0
frozen in syrup, Birds Eye, quick thaw pouch, 5 oz	120	0	0	0	0	0
Nectarine, 1 fruit (2½″)	70	N.A.	N.A.	<1	N.A.	0
Orange, 1 (2⅝″)	60	N.A.	N.A.	<1	N.A.	0
peel, 1 tbsp	0	0	0	0	0	0
Orange juice, fresh, 1 cup	110	N.A.	N.A.	<1	N.A.	0
canned, 1 cup	100	N.A.	N.A.	<1	N.A.	0

*Less than 2% U.S. RDA

Sodium (mg)	Potassium (mg)	Protein (g)	Carbohydrate (g)	Dietary fiber (g)	Sugars (g)	Calcium (% U.S. RDA)	Iron (% U.S. RDA)	Vitamin A (% U.S. RDA)	Vitamin C (% U.S. RDA)
5	55	<1	32	N.A.	36	*	2	*	100
0	260	<1	11	4.7	N.A.	2	2	15	280
45	N.A.	0	23	N.A.	N.A.	*	2	*	50
0	250	<1	11	0.4	8	2	2	2	120
0	35	<1	3	N.A.	N.A.	*	*	*	10
0	160	1	12	N.A.	2	6	6	*	140
0	80	<1	5	N.A.	N.A.	*	2	*	50
0	10	<1	1	N.A.	N.A.	*	*	*	15
0	20	<1	1	N.A.	N.A.	*	*	*	10
0	15	<1	1	N.A.	N.A.	*	*	*	6
0	70	<1	7	N.A.	N.A.	2	2	*	35
0	15	<1	1	N.A.	N.A.	*	*	*	8
0	10	0	1	N.A.	N.A.	*	*	*	2
0	320	1	35	2.3	N.A.	2	2	160	100
15	490	1	13	0.5	14	2	2	100	110
20	360	2	11	N.A.	N.A.	*	4	*	45
15	460	<1	16	0.9	N.A.	*	*	*	70
0	190	1	11	0.2	14	*	2	10	25
5	110	<1	24	N.A.	N.A.	*	4	6	150
50	2330	7	188	N.A.	N.A.	10	50	140	20
10	330	4	61	N.A.	N.A.	2	4	15	30
5	N.A.	1	31	1	16	*	2	6	45
0	290	1	16	N.A.	12	*	*	20	10
0	240	1	15	2.9	13	6	*	6	120
0	15	<1	2	N.A.	N.A.	*	*	*	15
0	500	2	26	N.A.	25	2	4	10	210
5	440	2	25	N.A.	N.A.	2	8	8	140

~ FRUITS & FRUIT JUICES	Calories	Saturated fat (g)	Polyunsat-urated fat (g)	Total fat (g)	Calories from fat	Choles-terol (mg)
frozen concentrate, diluted with 3 parts water, 1 cup	110	N.A.	N.A.	<1	N.A.	0
Oranges, mandarin, in light syrup, ½ cup	80	0	0	<1	N.A.	0
juice pack, ½ cup	45	0	0	0	0	0
Papaya, 1 (3½″ × 5⅛″)	120	N.A.	N.A.	<1	N.A.	0
Papaya nectar, canned, 1 cup	140	N.A.	N.A.	<1	N.A.	0
Passion fruit, 1 (1¼ oz)	18	N.A.	N.A.	<1	N.A.	0
Passion fruit juice, 1 cup	130	N.A.	N.A.	<1	N.A.	0
Peach, fresh, 2½″	35	N.A.	N.A.	<1	N.A.	0
canned water pack, 1 cup	60	N.A.	N.A.	<1	N.A.	0
juice pack, 1 cup	110	N.A.	N.A.	<1	N.A.	0
in light syrup, 1 cup	140	N.A.	N.A.	<1	N.A.	0
in heavy syrup, 1 cup	190	N.A.	N.A.	<1	N.A.	0
dehydrated (low-moisture), ½ cup	190	N.A.	N.A.	<1	N.A.	0
dried, ½ cup	190	<1	<1	<1	N.A.	0
frozen sweetened, sliced, 1 cup	240	N.A.	N.A.	<1	N.A.	0
Pear, fresh, 2½″ × 3½″	100	N.A.	N.A.	<1	N.A.	0
canned water pack, 1 cup	70	N.A.	N.A.	<1	N.A.	0
juice pack, 1 cup	120	N.A.	N.A.	<1	N.A.	0
in light syrup, 1 cup	140	N.A.	N.A.	<1	N.A.	0
in heavy syrup, 1 cup	190	N.A.	N.A.	<1	N.A.	0
dried, 1 cup	470	<1	<1	1	10	0
Pineapple, fresh, 1 cup pieces	80	N.A.	N.A.	<1	N.A.	0
canned water pack, 1 cup	80	N.A.	N.A.	<1	N.A.	0
juice pack, 1 cup	150	N.A.	N.A.	<1	N.A.	0
in light syrup, 1 cup	130	N.A.	N.A.	<1	N.A.	0
in heavy syrup, 1 cup	200	N.A.	N.A.	<1	N.A.	0
frozen chunks, sweetened, 1 cup	210	N.A.	N.A.	<1	N.A.	0

*Less than 2% U.S. RDA

Sodium (mg)	Potassium (mg)	Protein (g)	Carbohydrate (g)	Dietary fiber (g)	Sugars (g)	Calcium (% U.S. RDA)	Iron (% U.S. RDA)	Vitamin A (% U.S. RDA)	Vitamin C (% U.S. RDA)
0	470	2	27	N.A.	26	2	*	4	160
10	100	<1	20	N.A.	N.A.	*	2	20	40
5	170	<1	12	N.A.	N.A.	*	2	20	70
10	780	2	30	2.7	N.A.	8	2	120	310
15	80	<1	36	N.A.	N.A.	2	6	6	15
5	65	<1	4	0.1	N.A.	*	2	2	10
N.A.	N.A.	1	34	N.A.	N.A.	*	4	35	120
0	170	<1	10	0.5	8	*	*	10	10
10	240	1	15	N.A.	N.A.	*	6	25	10
10	320	2	29	1.2	43	2	6	20	15
15	240	1	37	N.A.	N.A.	*	6	20	10
15	240	1	51	N.A.	N.A.	*	4	15	10
5	780	3	48	N.A.	N.A.	2	20	15	10
5	800	3	49	4.2	N.A.	2	20	35	6
15	330	1	60	N.A.	N.A.	*	6	15	390
0	210	<1	25	4.2	17	2	2	*	10
5	130	<1	19	N.A.	15	*	4	*	4
10	240	<1	32	2.2	24	2	4	*	6
15	170	<1	38	N.A.	N.A.	*	4	*	4
15	170	<1	49	N.A.	39	*	4	*	4
10	960	3	125	N.A.	N.A.	6	25	*	20
0	180	<1	19	2.3	18	*	4	*	40
0	310	1	20	N.A.	N.A.	4	6	*	30
0	300	1	39	2	36	4	4	2	40
0	270	1	34	N.A.	N.A.	4	6	*	30
0	260	1	52	N.A.	N.A.	4	6	*	30
5	250	1	54	N.A.	N.A.	2	6	*	35

~ FRUITS & FRUIT JUICES	Calories	Saturated fat (g)	Polyunsat-urated fat (g)	Total fat (g)	Calories from fat	Choles-terol (mg)
Pineapple juice						
canned, 1 cup	140	N.A.	N.A.	<1	N.A.	0
frozen concentrate, diluted with 3 parts water, 1 cup	130	N.A.	N.A.	<1	N.A.	0
Plum, fresh, 2⅛″	35	N.A.	N.A.	<1	N.A.	0
purple, canned water pack, 1 cup	100	0	0	0	0	0
juice pack, 1 cup	150	0	0	0	0	0
in light syrup, 1 cup	160	N.A.	N.A.	<1	N.A.	0
in heavy syrup, 1 cup	230	N.A.	N.A.	<1	N.A.	0
Pomegranate, 1 (3⅜″ × 3¾″)	100	N.A.	N.A.	<1	N.A.	0
Prunes, canned in heavy syrup, 1 cup	250	N.A.	N.A.	<1	N.A.	0
dehydrated (low-moisture), 1 cup	450	0	<1	1	10	0
dried, 1 cup	390	N.A.	N.A.	<1	N.A.	0
Prune juice, canned, 1 cup	180	0	0	0	0	0
Quince, 1 (5¼ oz)	50	0	0	0	0	0
Raisins, 1 cup seedless, regular, golden	440	N.A.	N.A.	<1	N.A.	0
Raspberries, fresh, 1 cup	60	N.A.	N.A.	<1	N.A.	0
canned, heavy syrup, 1 cup	230	N.A.	N.A.	<1	N.A.	0
frozen sweetened, 1 cup	260	N.A.	N.A.	<1	N.A.	0
frozen in lite syrup, Birds Eye, quick thaw pouch, 5 oz	100	N.A.	N.A.	1	10	0
Rhubarb, fresh, 1 cup pieces	25	N.A.	N.A.	<1	N.A.	0
Strawberries, fresh, 1 cup	45	N.A.	N.A.	<1	N.A.	0
frozen halves in syrup, Birds Eye), 5 oz	120	0	0	0	0	0
in lite syrup	90	0	0	0	0	0
frozen sweetened, 1 cup whole or sliced	230	N.A.	N.A.	<1	N.A.	0
frozen unsweetened, 1 cup	50	N.A.	N.A.	<1	N.A.	0
Tangerine, 1 fresh (2⅜″)	35	N.A.	N.A.	<1	N.A.	0

*Less than 2% U.S. RDA

Sodium (mg)	Potassium (mg)	Protein (g)	Carbohydrate (g)	Dietary fiber (g)	Sugars (g)	Calcium (% U.S. RDA)	Iron (% U.S. RDA)	Vitamin A (% U.S. RDA)	Vitamin C (% U.S. RDA)
0	330	<1	34	N.A.	31	4	4	*	45
0	340	1	32	N.A.	N.A.	2	6	*	50
0	115	<1	9	1.1	5	*	*	4	10
0	310	1	27	N.A.	N.A.	*	2	45	10
0	390	1	38	1	N.A.	2	6	50	10
50	230	1	41	N.A.	N.A.	2	15	15	2
50	230	1	60	N.A.	N.A.	2	15	15	2
5	400	2	26	5.2	N.A.	*	4	N.A.	15
5	530	2	65	N.A.	N.A.	4	6	35	10
5	1400	5	118	N.A.	N.A.	10	30	45	*
5	1200	4	101	10.9	N.A.	8	25	60	10
10	710	2	45	N.A.	34	4	20	*	20
0	180	<1	14	N.A.	N.A.	*	4	*	25
15	1090	5	115	3	98	8	20	*	8
0	190	1	14	5.8	N.A.	2	4	4	50
10	240	2	60	N.A.	N.A.	2	8	2	35
1	290	2	65	N.A.	N.A.	4	10	2	70
0	140	1	25	N.A.	20	2	2	2	40
5	350	1	6	2	N.A.	10	2	2	15
0	250	1	10	2.8	9	2	4	*	140
0	190	1	30	N.A.	N.A.	*	4	*	110
5	190	1	22	N.A.	21	*	2	*	110
5	250	1	60	N.A.	N.A.	2	10	*	180
0	220	<1	14	N.A.	N.A.	2	8	*	100
0	130	<1	9	N.A.	N.A.	*	*	15	45

∿ GRAINS

∿ PASTA

∿ & FLOUR

∿ *Prepared rice and pasta side dishes are listed under "Entrees and Side Dishes." Grains are a major source of fiber, both soluble and insoluble; simple sugars are negligible in basic grain products.*

∿ GRAINS, PASTA & FLOUR

	Calories	Saturated fat (g)	Polyunsaturated fat (g)	Total fat (g)	Calories from fat	Cholesterol (mg)
Baking powder, 1 tsp	4	0	0	0	N.A.	0
low sodium, 1 tsp	8	0	0	0	0	N.A.
Baking soda, 1 tsp	N.A.	N.A.	N.A.	N.A.	N.A.	N.A.
Barley, pearled, ½ cup cooked	100	0	<1	<1	N.A.	0
Buckwheat groats (kasha), ½ cup cooked	90	<1	<1	<1	N.A.	0
Bulgur, ½ cup cooked	80	0	0	<1	N.A.	0
Cornmeal, whole grain, 1 cup	440	<1	2	4	35	0
degermed, 1 cup	510	<1	1	2	18	0
self-rising bolted, 1 cup	410	<1	2	4	35	0
self-rising degermed, 1 cup	490	<1	1	2	18	0
Cornstarch, 1 cup	490	0	0	0	N.A.	0
1 tbsp	30	0	0	0	N.A.	0
Couscous, ½ cup cooked	100	0	0	<1	N.A.	0
Cream of tartar, 1 tbsp	8	0	0	0	0	N.A.
Farina (see Breakfast Cereals)						
Flour						
arrowroot, 1 cup	460	0	0	<1	N.A.	0
bread, white, 1 cup	500	<1	1	2	18	0
buckwheat, whole groat, ½ cup	200	<1	<1	2	18	0
cake, white, 1 cup	400	<1	<1	<1	N.A.	0
corn, whole grain, 1 cup	420	<1	2	5	45	0
oat blend, Gold Medal, 1 cup (4 oz)	390	N.A.	N.A.	3	25	N.A.
potato, 1 cup	630	<1	<1	1	10	0
rice, brown, 1 cup	570	<1	2	4	35	0
white, 1 cup	580	<1	<1	2	18	0
rye, dark, 1 cup	420	<1	2	3	25	0
medium, 1 cup	360	<1	<1	2	18	0
light, 1 cup	370	<1	<1	1	10	0
soy flour, meal (see Legumes & Seeds)						

*Less than 2% U.S. RDA

Sodium (mg)	Potassium (mg)	Protein (g)	Carbohy-drate (g)	Dietary fiber (g)	Calcium (% U.S. RDA)	Iron (% U.S. RDA)	Vitamin A (% U.S. RDA)	Vitamin C (% U.S. RDA)
430	0	<1	0	N.A.	25	*	*	*
0	N.A.	0	2	N.A.	*	*	*	*
1100	N.A.	N.A.	N.A.	N.A.	N.A.	N.A.	N.A.	N.A.
0	75	2	22	N.A.	*	8	*	*
0	90	3	20	N.A.	*	6	*	*
5	60	3	17	N.A.	*	6	*	*
45	350	10	94	13.4	*	30	10	*
5	220	12	107	7.2	*	40	10	*
1520	310	10	86	N.A.	45	45	*	*
1860	240	12	103	N.A.	50	45	*	*
10	0	<1	117	1.2	*	4	N.A.	*
0	0	0	7	0.1	*	*	N.A.	*
0	50	3	21	N.A.	*	2	*	*
690	360	2	0	N.A.	*	*	*	*
0	15	<1	113	4.4	6	2	*	*
0	135	16	99	N.A.	2	40	N.A.	*
N.A.	350	8	42	1.6	2	15	*	*
0	115	9	85	N.A.	*	50	N.A.	*
5	370	8	90	15.7	*	20	*	*
0	210	14	81	4	2	20	*	*
60	2840	14	143	N.A.	6	210	*	60
10	460	11	121	7.3	*	20	*	*
0	120	9	127	3.8	*	4	*	*
0	930	18	88	N.A.	8	60	*	*
0	350	10	79	14.9	2	15	*	*
0	240	9	82	14.9	2	10	*	*

~ GRAINS, PASTA & FLOUR	Calories	Saturated fat (g)	Polyunsat-urated fat (g)	Total fat (g)	Calories from fat	Choles-terol (mg)
triticale, whole grain, 1 cup	440	<1	1	2	18	0
white, all-purpose, 1 cup	460	<1	<1	1	10	0
self-rising, 1 cup	440	<1	<1	1	10	0
whole wheat, 1 cup	410	<1	<1	2	18	0
whole wheat blend, Gold Medal, 1 cup	380	N.A.	N.A.	2	18	N.A.
Grits (see Breakfast Cereals)						
Hominy, canned white or yellow, ½ cup	60	<1	<1	<1	N.A.	0
Kasha (see Buckwheat groats, above)						
Macaroni (see Pasta, below)						
Millet, ½ cup cooked	140	<1	<1	1	10	0
Noodles						
cellophane (long rice), ½ cup dry	250	0	0	0	0	0
chow mein, 1 cup	240	2	8	14	130	0
egg, ½ cup cooked	110	<1	<1	1	10	26
spinach, ½ cup	110	<1	<1	1	10	26
Oat Bran (see Breakfast Cereals)						
Oatmeal (see Breakfast Cereals)						
Pasta						
fresh refrigerated, 2 oz cooked, plain or spinach	80	<1	<1	<1	N.A.	19
regular dry, ½ cup cooked	100	<1	<1	<1	N.A.	0
protein-fortified, ½ cup	100	<1	<1	<1	N.A.	0
vegetable pasta, ½ cup	90	0	0	0	0	0
whole wheat, ½ cup	90	0	<1	<1	N.A.	0
Pasta side dishes (see Entrees & Side Dishes)						
Polenta, Fantastic Foods, ½ cup (⅙ pkg)	110	N.A.	N.A.	2	18	N.A.

*Less than 2% U.S. RDA

Sodium (mg)	Potassium (mg)	Protein (g)	Carbohy-drate (g)	Dietary fiber (g)	Calcium (% U.S. RDA)	Iron (% U.S. RDA)	Vitamin A (% U.S. RDA)	Vitamin C (% U.S. RDA)
0	610	17	95	19	4	25	*	*
0	135	13	95	3.4	*	40	N.A.	*
1590	160	12	93	N.A.	40	40	N.A.	*
5	490	16	87	15.1	4	30	N.A.	*
0	340	14	84	8	2	25	*	*
170	5	1	11	N.A.	*	4	*	*
0	75	4	28	N.A.	*	6	*	*
5	5	<1	60	N.A.	*	10	*	*
200	55	4	26	1.8	*	15	*	*
5	25	4	20	1.8	*	8	*	*
10	30	4	19	4	*	6	*	*
0	20	3	14	N.A.	*	4	N.A.	*
0	20	3	20	1.1	*	6	N.A.	*
0	25	5	18	1	*	2	N.A.	*
0	20	3	18	5	*	2	*	*
0	30	4	19	5.5	*	4	N.A.	*
250	N.A.	3	18	N.A.	N.A.	N.A.	N.A.	N.A.

~ GRAINS, PASTA & FLOUR	Calories	Saturated fat (g)	Polyunsaturated fat (g)	Total fat (g)	Calories from fat	Cholesterol (mg)
Popcorn (see Crackers, Chips, and Other Snacks)						
Ramen noodles, La Choy, 1 cup, beef, chicken	210	1	3	8	70	0
Rice						
brown, ½ cup cooked	110	<1	<1	<1	N.A.	0
instant, Minute Rice, ½ cup	120	N.A.	N.A.	1	10	0
white, ½ cup cooked	130	<1	<1	<1	N.A.	0
parboiled, ½ cup cooked	100	<1	<1	<1	N.A.	0
instant, Minute Rice, ½ cup, no butter or salt	90	0	0	0	0	0
flavored mixes, Minute Rice, ½ cup	150	N.A.	N.A.	4	35	10
wild rice, ½ cup cooked	80	0	<1	<1	N.A.	0
Uncle Ben's long grain and, ½ cup, original flavor	100	0	0	0	0	N.A.
fast-cooking	100	N.A.	N.A.	1	10	N.A.
garden vegetable	130	N.A.	N.A.	1	10	N.A.
Rice bran, Uncle Ben's "Rite-Bran," ½ cup	100	N.A.	N.A.	9	80	N.A.
Rice side dishes (see Entrees & Side Dishes)						
Semolina, ½ cup	300	<1	<1	<1	N.A.	0
Spaghetti (see Pasta, above)						
Tabbouleh, Fantastic Foods, ½ cup	160	N.A.	N.A.	10	90	N.A.
Tapioca, quick cooking, 2 tbsp	60	0	0	0	0	N.A.
Wheat bran, crude, ½ cup	70	<1	<1	1	10	0
Wheat germ, crude, 1 cup	410	2	7	11	100	0
toasted, 1 cup	430	2	8	12	110	0
Wild rice (see Rice, above)						

*Less than 2% U.S. RDA

Sodium (mg)	Potassium (mg)	Protein (g)	Carbohydrate (g)	Dietary fiber (g)	Calcium (% U.S. RDA)	Iron (% U.S. RDA)	Vitamin A (% U.S. RDA)	Vitamin C (% U.S. RDA)
800	40	6	31	4	*	10	*	*
5	40	3	23	1.7	*	2	*	*
5	N.A.	3	26	N.A.	*	2	*	*
0	40	3	29	0.5	*	8	N.A.	*
0	35	2	22	0.4	*	6	*	*
0	0	2	20	N.A.	*	4	*	*
630	35	3	25	N.A.	*	6	2	*
0	85	3	18	0.6	*	4	*	*
500	N.A.	3	22	N.A.	2	6	*	2
410	N.A.	3	21	N.A.	*	6	*	*
610	N.A.	3	27	N.A.	15	4	*	2
5	N.A.	5	10	9	4	15	*	*
0	160	11	61	3.3	*	25	*	*
250	N.A.	2	17	N.A.	N.A.	N.A.	N.A.	N.A.
0	0	<1	15	N.A.	*	*	*	*
0	360	5	19	12.7	2	20	*	*
15	1030	27	60	17.3	4	50	N.A.	*
0	1070	33	56	14.6	6	70	N.A.	10

~ GRAINS, PASTA & FLOUR	Calories	Saturated fat (g)	Polyunsaturated fat (g)	Total fat (g)	Calories from fat	Cholesterol (mg)
Yeast						
active dry, Fleischmann's, regular or rapid rise, 1 packet	20	0	0	0	0	N.A.
compressed, 1 cube	15	0	0	0	0	N.A.
nutritional, 1 oz	80	N.A.	N.A.	<1	N.A.	N.A.

*Less than 2% U.S. RDA

Sodium (mg)	Potassium (mg)	Protein (g)	Carbohy-drate (g)	Dietary fiber (g)	Calcium (% U.S. RDA)	Iron (% U.S. RDA)	Vitamin A (% U.S. RDA)	Vitamin C (% U.S. RDA)
10	150	3	3	N.A.	N.A.	N.A.	N.A.	N.A.
5	100	2	2	N.A.	N.A.	N.A.	N.A.	N.A.
0	580	11	11	N.A.	10	35	*	*

∾ LEGUMES

∾ (Beans, Nuts)

∾ & SEEDS

∾ Prepared dishes are listed under "Entrees & Side Dishes." Legumes are a major source of fiber, both soluble and insoluble. Some soy products are listed with other foods with which they might be compared—e.g., tofutti is listed with "Dairy Products & Eggs."

～ LEGUMES & SEEDS

	Calories	Saturated fat (g)	Polyunsat-urated fat (g)	Total fat (g)	Calories from fat	Choles-terol (mg)
Almond paste, 1 oz	130	<1	2	8	70	0
Beans						
adzuki, cooked, ½ cup	150	N.A.	N.A.	<1	N.A.	0
canned sweetened, ½ cup	350	N.A.	N.A.	<1	N.A.	0
black, ½ cup cooked	110	<1	<1	<1	N.A.	0
canned, Progresso, ½ cup	90	N.A.	N.A.	<1	N.A.	0
instant, Fantastic Foods, ½ cup	160	N.A.	N.A.	2	18	N.A.
black turtle soup, ½ cup cooked	120	<1	<1	<1	N.A.	0
canned, ½ cup	110	<1	<1	<1	N.A.	0
black-eyed peas (cowpeas), ½ cup cooked	100	<1	<1	<1	N.A.	0
canned, ½ cup	90	<1	<1	<1	N.A.	0
chick-peas, ½ cup cooked	130	<1	1	2	18	0
canned, Progresso, ½ cup	120	N.A.	N.A.	1	10	0
cranberry, ½ cup cooked	120	<1	<1	<1	N.A.	0
garbanzos (see chick-peas, above)						
great northern, ½ cup cooked	100	<1	<1	<1	N.A.	0
canned, Green Giant, ½ cup)	80	N.A.	N.A.	1	10	0
kidney, ½ cup cooked	110	<1	<1	<1	N.A.	0
canned, Progresso, ½ cup	100	N.A.	N.A.	<1	N.A.	0
lima, ½ cup cooked, large white	110	<1	<1	<1	N.A.	0
canned, ½ cup	100	<1	<1	<1	N.A.	0
baby limas, ½ cup cooked	120	<1	<1	<1	N.A.	0
navy, ½ cup cooked	130	<1	<1	<1	N.A.	0
canned, ½ cup	150	<1	<1	<1	N.A.	0
pinto, ½ cup cooked	120	<1	<1	<1	N.A.	0
canned, Progresso, ½ cup	110	N.A.	N.A.	<1	N.A.	0

*Less than 2% U.S. RDA

Sodium (mg)	Potassium (mg)	Protein (g)	Carbohy-drate (g)	Dietary fiber (g)	Calcium (% U.S. RDA)	Iron (% U.S. RDA)	Vitamin A (% U.S. RDA)	Vitamin C (% U.S. RDA)
0	180	3	12	N.A.	6	6	*	*
10	610	9	29	N.A.	4	15	*	*
320	180	6	81	N.A.	4	10	N.A.	N.A.
0	310	8	20	N.A.	2	10	*	*
480	290	9	19	6.5	4	10	*	*
400	N.A.	10	28	N.A.	N.A.	N.A.	N.A.	N.A.
0	400	8	22	N.A.	6	15	*	*
460	370	7	20	N.A.	4	15	*	6
0	240	7	18	N.A.	2	15	*	*
360	210	6	16	4.7	2	8	*	6
5	240	7	22	N.A.	4	15	*	*
390	130	9	22	6	4	4	*	*
0	340	8	22	5.4	4	10	*	*
0	340	7	19	N.A.	6	15	*	*
290	150	6	18	5	10	10	*	*
0	360	8	20	N.A.	2	15	*	*
420	220	9	21	7	4	10	*	*
0	480	7	20	3.1	*	15	*	*
400	260	6	18	N.A.	2	15	*	*
0	370	7	21	4	2	15	*	*
0	340	8	24	6.5	6	15	*	*
590	380	10	27	N.A.	6	15	*	*
0	400	7	22	N.A.	4	15	*	2
410	200	8	21	6.5	4	8	*	*

~ LEGUMES & SEEDS	Calories	Saturated fat (g)	Polyunsaturated fat (g)	Total fat (g)	Calories from fat	Cholesterol (mg)
canned picante style, Green Giant, ½ cup	100	N.A.	N.A.	1	10	0
frozen, ⅓ of 10-oz pkg	150	<1	<1	<1	N.A.	0
see also Refried beans, below						
soybeans, ½ cup cooked	150	1	4	8	70	0
roasted, ½ cup	410	3	12	22	200	0
dry roasted, ½ cup	390	3	11	19	170	0
Beans, canned prepared						
plain or vegetarian, ½ cup	120	<1	<1	<1	N.A.	0
with franks, ½ cup	180	3	1	8	70	8
with pork and tomato sauce, ½ cup	120	<1	<1	1	10	9
Cashew butter, 1 tbsp (½ oz) (salted has 100 mg sodium)	90	2	1	8	70	0
Chili with beans (see Entrees & Side Dishes)						
Coconut milk, fresh, 1 cup	550	51	<1	57	510	0
Falafel, 1 patty, ½–⅔ oz (2¼" diameter)	60	<1	<1	3	25	0
Hummus, ⅓ cup	140	1	3	7	60	0
Lentils, ½ cup cooked	120	<1	<1	<1	N.A.	0
Longrice (mung bean), ½ cup dehydrated	250	<1	<1	<1	N.A.	0
Miso, ½ cup	280	1	5	8	70	0
Natto, ½ cup	190	1	6	10	90	0
Nuts						
almonds, 1 oz fresh (about 24 nuts)	170	1	3	15	140	0
1 cup whole (about 5 oz)	850	7	16	76	680	0
1 cup sliced (about 3⅔ oz)	610	5	11	55	500	0
dry roasted, 1 oz	170	1	3	15	140	0

*Less than 2% U.S. RDA

Sodium (mg)	Potassium (mg)	Protein (g)	Carbohy-drate (g)	Dietary fiber (g)	Calcium (% U.S. RDA)	Iron (% U.S. RDA)	Vitamin A (% U.S. RDA)	Vitamin C (% U.S. RDA)
580	270	7	21	6	4	8	6	*
N.A.	N.A.	9	29	N.A.	4	15	*	*
0	440	14	9	N.A.	8	30	*	2
140	1260	30	29	N.A.	10	25	4	4
0	1170	34	28	N.A.	25	25	*	6
500	380	6	26	4.4	6	2	*	N.A.
550	300	9	20	4	6	10	4	4
550	380	7	24	3.7	8	25	4	6
0	85	3	4	N.A.	*	6	*	*
35	630	6	13	N.A.	4	25	*	10
50	100	2	5	N.A.	*	*	*	*
200	140	4	17	N.A.	4	8	*	10
0	370	9	20	5.2	*	20	*	2
5	5	<1	60	N.A.	*	10	*	*
5030	230	16	39	3.9	10	25	2	*
5	640	16	13	N.A.	20	50	*	20
0	210	6	5	1.7	*	6	*	*
15	1090	30	27	8.7	4	35	*	*
10	790	21	20	6.3	2	25	*	*
0	220	5	7	N.A.	8	8	*	*

~ LEGUMES & SEEDS	Calories	Saturated fat (g)	Polyunsaturated fat (g)	Total fat (g)	Calories from fat	Cholesterol (mg)
honey roasted, Planters, 1 oz (unsalted contains 180 mg sodium)	170	1	3	13	120	0
oil roasted, 1 oz (about 22) (unsalted contains 0 mg sodium)	180	2	3	16	140	0
beechnuts, 1 oz dried	160	2	6	14	130	0
Brazil nuts, 1 oz (about 6 large)	190	5	7	19	170	0
butternuts, 1 oz dried	170	<1	12	16	140	0
cashews, 1 oz dry roasted	160	3	2	13	120	0
oil roasted (about 18 medium) (unsalted contains 5 mg sodium)	160	3	2	14	130	0
chestnuts, Chinese, 1 oz roasted	70	<1	<1	<1	N.A.	0
European, 1 oz roasted (about 3½ nuts)	70	<1	<1	<1	N.A.	0
coconut, 1 cup fresh shredded (2¾ oz)	280	24	<1	27	240	0
dried unsweetened, ⅓ cup (1 oz)	190	16	<1	18	160	0
dried sweetened, canned flaked, 1 cup (2¾ oz)	340	22	<1	24	220	0
dried sweetened, shredded, 1 cup (3¼ oz)	470	29	<1	33	300	0
filberts, 1 oz dried (¼ cup)	180	1	2	18	160	0
dry or oil roasted, 1 oz	190	1	2	19	170	0
formulated nuts (wheat based) (see Crackers, Chips & Other Snacks)						
hazelnuts (see filberts, above)						
macadamia, 1 oz (scant ¼ cup), dried, oil roasted (unsalted contains 0 mg sodium)	200	3	<1	22	200	0

*Less than 2% U.S. RDA

Sodium (mg)	Potassium (mg)	Protein (g)	Carbohydrate (g)	Dietary fiber (g)	Calcium (% U.S. RDA)	Iron (% U.S. RDA)	Vitamin A (% U.S. RDA)	Vitamin C (% U.S. RDA)
220	170	5	9	N.A.	4	4	*	*
220	190	6	5	N.A.	6	8	*	*
N.A.	N.A.	2	10	N.A.	N.A.	*	N.A.	N.A.
0	170	4	4	N.A.	6	6	*	*
0	120	7	3	N.A.	*	8	N.A.	N.A.
0	160	4	9	N.A.	*	10	*	*
180	150	5	8	N.A.	*	8	*	*
0	135	1	15	N.A.	*	2	*	N.A.
0	170	<1	15	3.7	*	2	*	10
15	290	3	12	6.6	*	15	*	4
10	150	2	7	4.7	*	6	*	*
15	250	3	32	N.A.	*	10	*	*
240	310	3	44	N.A.	*	10	*	*
0	125	4	4	2	6	6	*	*
0	130	4	5	N.A.	6	6	N.A.	N.A.
75	100	2	4	N.A.	*	4	*	*

LEGUMES & SEEDS	Calories	Saturated fat (g)	Polyunsat-urated fat (g)	Total fat (g)	Calories from fat	Choles-terol (mg)
mixed nuts with peanuts, 1 oz dry roasted (¼ cup) (unsalted has 0 mg sodium)	170	2	3	15	140	0
oil roasted, 1 oz (unsalted has 0 mg sodium)	180	2	4	16	140	0
oil roasted, no peanuts, 1 oz (unsalted has 0 mg sodium)	180	3	3	16	140	0
peanuts, 1 oz plain (3 tbsp)	160	2	4	14	130	0
oil roasted, 1 oz (3 tbsp) (dry roasted contains 230 mg sodium; un-salted, both con-tain 0 mg sodium)	160	2	4	14	130	0
pecans, 1 oz (¼ cup)	190	2	5	19	170	0
dry roasted, 1 oz (un-salted contains 0 mg sodium)	190	2	5	18	160	0
oil roasted, 1 oz (unsalted contains 0 mg sodium)	200	2	5	20	180	0
pine nuts, 1 oz (2¾ tbsp)	150	2	6	14	130	0
pistachios, 1 oz (¼ cup)	160	2	2	14	130	0
dry roasted, 1 oz	170	2	2	15	140	0
walnuts, black, 1 oz (¼ cup)	170	1	11	16	140	0
English, 1 oz (¼ cup)	180	2	11	18	160	0
Nut topping, Planters, 1 oz	180	2	5	16	140	0
Peanut butter, chunky or smooth, 2 tbsp (sodium-free varieties contain 0 mg sodium)	190	3	5	16	140	0
Peas, green (see Vegetables)						
Pumpkin/squash seeds, 1 oz roasted (½ cup)	130	1	3	6	50	0
Refried beans, Old El Paso, ¼ cup, with bacon	100	1	0	4	35	6

*Less than 2% U.S. RDA

Sodium (mg)	Potassium (mg)	Protein (g)	Carbohydrate (g)	Dietary fiber (g)	Calcium (% U.S. RDA)	Iron (% U.S. RDA)	Vitamin A (% U.S. RDA)	Vitamin C (% U.S. RDA)
190	170	5	7	N.A.	2	8	*	*
190	170	5	6	N.A.	4	6	*	*
200	150	4	6	N.A.	4	4	*	*
5	200	7	5	2.1	2	8	*	*
120	190	7	5	N.A.	2	4	*	*
0	110	2	5	N.A.	*	4	*	*
200	105	2	6	N.A.	*	4	N.A.	N.A.
210	100	2	5	N.A.	*	4	N.A.	N.A.
0	170	7	4	N.A.	*	15	N.A.	N.A.
0	310	6	7	N.A.	4	15	*	*
0	280	4	8	N.A.	2	6	N.A.	N.A.
0	150	7	3	1.6	*	6	*	*
0	140	4	5	1.3	2	4	*	*
0	170	5	6	N.A.	*	2	*	*
160	240	8	7	0.9	*	4	*	*
5	260	5	15	N.A.	*	6	N.A.	N.A.
190	250	6	12	5	2	6	*	6

~ LEGUMES & SEEDS	Calories	Saturated fat (g)	Polyunsaturated fat (g)	Total fat (g)	Calories from fat	Cholesterol (mg)
with cheese	35	1	0	1	10	2
with jalapeños	30	0	0	1	10	1
vegetarian	70	N.A.	N.A.	1	10	0
Sesame seeds, 1 tbsp	50	<1	2	4	35	0
Simulated meat, bacon, 1 strip (¼ oz)	25	<1	1	2	18	0
meat extender, 1 cup	280	<1	2	3	25	0
sausage, 1 link (1 oz)	60	<1	2	5	45	0
sausage, 1 patty (1⅓ oz)	100	1	4	7	60	0
see also specific listings under Meat, Poultry, Fish & Simulated Meats *and* Entrees & Side Dishes						
Soy cheese , Soyco, 1 oz, all varieties	70	1	<1	5	45	0
Soy flour, full-fat, 1 cup	370	3	10	18	160	0
defatted, 1 cup	330	<1	<1	1	10	0
Soy meal, defatted, 1 cup	410	<1	1	3	25	0
Soy milk, ½ cup	40	<1	1	2	18	0
powdered Soyamel, Worthington Foods, 1 cup prepared	130	1	2	7	60	0
Soy sauce (*see* Condiments)						
Split peas, ½ cup cooked	120	<1	<1	<1	N.A.	0
Sunflower seeds, 1 oz (3 tbsp)	160	2	9	14	130	0
dry roasted, 1 oz (3½ tbsp)	170	2	9	14	130	0
oil roasted, 1 oz (3 tbsp)	180	2	11	16	140	0
Tahini (sesame butter), 1 tbsp	90	1	3	7	60	0
Tempeh, ½ cup	170	<1	4	6	50	0
Three bean salad (*see* Vegetables)						
Tofu, fresh firm, ½ cup† (4½ oz)	180	2	6	11	100	0

*Less than 2% U.S. RDA
†If calcium sulfate is used, fresh firm tofu contains 90% U.S. RDA for calcium, and fresh regular tofu contains 45% U.S. RDA for calcium.

Sodium (mg)	Potassium (mg)	Protein (g)	Carbohy-drate (g)	Dietary fiber (g)	Calcium (% U.S. RDA)	Iron (% U.S. RDA)	Vitamin A (% U.S. RDA)	Vitamin C (% U.S. RDA)
280	80	2	4	2	2	2	*	*
270	85	1	4	2	*	2	*	*
590	320	6	15	5	2	15	*	*
0	40	2	2	0.8	8	8	*	*
115	15	<1	<1	N.A.	*	*	*	*
10	N.A.	34	34	N.A.	20	10	*	*
220	60	5	2	N.A.	*	6	4	*
340	90	7	4	N.A.	2	10	4	*
140	N.A.	7	<1	N.A.	20	*	6	*
10	2140	29	30	N.A.	20	35	2	*
20	2380	47	38	N.A.	25	60	*	*
0	3040	55	49	N.A.	30	110	*	*
15	170	3	2	N.A.	*	4	*	*
210	270	7	10	N.A.	35	6	10	2
0	360	8	21	3.1	*	8	*	*
0	200	7	5	1.5	4	15	*	N.A.
0	240	6	7	N.A.	2	8	N.A.	N.A.
0	135	6	4	N.A.	*	15	N.A.	*
10	60	3	4	N.A.	6	2	N.A.	*
5	310	16	14	N.A.	8	15	10	*
15	300	20	5	N.A.	25	90	4	*

~ LEGUMES & SEEDS	Calories	Saturated fat (g)	Polyunsaturated fat (g)	Total fat (g)	Calories from fat	Cholesterol (mg)
fresh regular, ½ cup†	90	<1	3	6	50	0
salted and fermented, 1 block (⅓ oz)	14	<1	<1	<1	N.A.	0
Tofutti, frozen soy dessert (see Dairy Products & Eggs)						

*Less than 2% U.S. RDA
†If calcium sulfate is used, fresh firm tofu contains 90% U.S. RDA for calcium, and fresh regular tofu contains 45% U.S. RDA for calcium.

Sodium (mg)	Potassium (mg)	Protein (g)	Carbohy-drate (g)	Dietary Fiber (g)	Calcium (% U.S. RDA)	Iron (% U.S. RDA)	Vitamin A (% U.S. RDA)	Vitamin C (% U.S. RDA)
10	150	10	2	0.6	15	45	2	*
320	10	<1	<1	N.A.	*	*	N.A.	N.A.

~ MEAT

~ POULTRY

~ FISH

~ & SIMULATED MEATS

~ *This section is divided into beef and veal, fish and seafood, lamb, pork, poultry, sausages and luncheon meat, simulated products, and variety meats. Listings are for basic cuts and preparations. Meat-based entrees and dinners are listed under "Entrees & Side Dishes." Meat and fish are not sources of fiber and sugar.*

	Calories	Saturated fat (g)	Polyunsaturated fat (g)	Total fat (g)	Calories from fat	Cholesterol (mg)
Beef breakfast strips, 3 slices cooked	150	5	<1	12	110	40
Brisket, fresh, braised, lean and fat, 3 oz	330	11	1	28	250	79
lean only, 3 oz	210	4	<1	11	100	79
Corned beef brisket, 3 oz cooked	210	5	<1	16	140	83
canned, 3 oz	210	5	<1	13	120	72
Dried beef, 1 oz	45	<1	<1	1	10	N.A.
Beef roast						
chuck (pot) roast, braised, lean and fat, 3 oz	300	9	<1	22	200	84
lean only, 3 oz	200	3	<1	9	80	85
rib roast, lean and fat, 3 oz	320	11	1	27	240	72
lean only, 3 oz	200	5	<1	12	110	68
round, bottom, braised, lean and fat, 3 oz	220	5	<1	13	120	81
lean only, 3 oz	190	3	<1	8	70	81
round, eye of, roasted, lean and fat, 3 oz	210	5	<1	12	110	62
lean only, 3 oz	160	2	<1	6	50	59
round, top, roasted, lean and fat, 3 oz	180	3	<1	8	70	72
lean only, 3 oz	160	2	<1	5	45	72
Ground beef						
regular (no more than 30% fat by weight), 4 oz raw	350	12	1	30	270	96
broiled, well-done, 3 oz (yield from 4 oz raw)	250	7	<1	17	150	86
lean (chuck), 4 oz raw	300	9	1	23	210	85
broiled, well-done, 3 oz (yield from 4 oz raw)	240	6	<1	15	140	86

*Less than 2% U.S. RDA

Sodium (mg)	Potassium (mg)	Protein (g)	Carbohydrate (g)	Calcium (% U.S. RDA)	Iron (% U.S. RDA)	Vitamin A (% U.S. RDA)	Vitamin C (% U.S. RDA)
770	140	11	<1	N.A.	8	N.A.	20
50	200	20	0	*	15	N.A.	*
60	240	25	0	*	15	N.A.	*
960	125	15	<1	*	10	N.A.	25
860	115	23	0	N.A.	10	*	2
980	125	8	<1	*	8	N.A.	N.A.
50	210	23	0	*	20	N.A.	*
55	250	28	0	*	20	N.A.	*
55	250	19	0	*	10	N.A.	*
65	320	23	0	*	15	N.A.	*
45	250	25	0	*	20	N.A.	*
45	260	27	0	*	20	N.A.	*
50	310	23	0	*	10	N.A.	*
50	340	25	0	*	10	N.A.	*
50	370	26	0	*	15	N.A.	*
50	380	27	0	*	15	N.A.	*
75	260	19	0	*	15	N.A.	*
80	280	23	0	*	15	N.A.	*
80	300	20	0	*	15	N.A.	*
75	300	24	0	*	15	N.A.	*

~ BEEF & VEAL

	Calories	Saturated fat (g)	Polyunsaturated fat (g)	Total fat (g)	Calories from fat	Cholesterol (mg)
extra lean (round, sirloin), 4 oz raw	270	8	<1	19	170	78
broiled, well-done, 3 oz (yield from 4 oz raw)	230	5	<1	13	120	84
Shank, simmered, lean and fat, 3 oz	210	4	<1	10	90	67
lean only, 3 oz	170	2	<1	5	45	66
Short ribs, braised, lean and fat, 3 oz	400	15	1	36	320	80
lean only, 3 oz	250	7	<1	15	140	79
Steak						
porterhouse, broiled, lean and fat, 3 oz	250	8	<1	18	160	70
lean only, 3 oz	190	4	<1	9	80	68
round, top, broiled, lean and fat, 3 oz	180	3	<1	8	70	72
lean only, 3 oz	160	2	<1	5	45	72
sirloin, broiled, lean and fat, 3 oz	240	6	<1	15	140	77
lean only, 3 oz	180	3	<1	7	60	76
T-bone, broiled, lean and fat, 3 oz	280	9	<1	21	190	71
lean only, 3 oz	180	4	<1	9	80	68
tenderloin, broiled, lean and fat, 3 oz	230	6	<1	15	140	73
lean only, 3 oz	170	3	<1	8	70	72
Steak-umm, frozen, 2 oz	180	N.A.	N.A.	16	140	N.A.
Veal						
breast, braised or stewed, 3 oz	260	9	N.A.	18	160	N.A.
chuck, braised, pot-roasted, or stewed, 3 oz	200	5	N.A.	11	100	N.A.
loin, braised or broiled, 3 oz	200	6	N.A.	11	100	N.A.
rib roast, roasted, 3 oz	230	7	N.A.	14	130	N.A.

*Less than 2% U.S. RDA

Sodium (mg)	Potassium (mg)	Protein (g)	Carbohy-drate (g)	Calcium (% U.S. RDA)	Iron (% U.S. RDA)	Vitamin A (% U.S. RDA)	Vitamin C (% U.S. RDA)
75	320	21	0	*	15	N.A.	*
70	310	24	0	*	15	N.A.	*
50	360	27	0	2	20	N.A.	*
55	380	29	0	2	20	N.A.	*
45	190	18	0	*	15	N.A.	*
50	270	26	0	*	20	N.A.	*
50	300	21	0	*	15	N.A.	*
55	350	24	0	*	20	N.A.	*
50	370	26	0	*	15	N.A.	*
50	380	27	0	*	15	N.A.	*
55	310	23	0	*	15	N.A.	*
55	340	26	0	*	20	N.A.	*
50	290	20	0	*	15	N.A.	*
55	350	24	0	*	15	N.A.	*
50	320	22	0	*	20	N.A.	*
55	360	24	0	*	20	N.A.	*
50	105	9	0	*	6	*	*
40	180	22	0	*	20	N.A.	N.A.
40	190	24	0	*	20	N.A.	N.A.
55	250	22	0	*	20	N.A.	N.A.
55	260	23	0	*	20	N.A.	N.A.

	Calories	Saturated fat (g)	Polyunsat-urated fat (g)	Total fat (g)	Calories from fat	Choles-terol (mg)
round with rump, braised or broiled, 3 oz	180	5	N.A.	9	80	N.A.
Abalone, floured and fried, 3 oz	160	1	1	6	50	80
Anchovy, fresh raw, 3 oz	110	1	1	4	35	N.A.
canned in oil, drained, 5 anchovies (¾ oz)	40	<1	<1	2	18	N.A.
Bass, 2¾ oz raw (fillet from 1-lb whole fish)	90	<1	<1	3	25	60
Carp, 6 oz broiled or baked (1 fillet from 3-lb whole fish)	280	2	3	12	110	143
Catfish, 3 oz breaded and fried (1 fillet from 1-lb whole fish)	200	3	3	12	110	70
Caviar, black and red, 1 tbsp	40	N.A.	N.A.	3	25	94
Clam broth, 3 oz canned	2	0	0	0	0	N.A.
Clams, raw or steamed, 9 large or 20 small (6⅓ oz raw)	130	<1	<1	2	18	60
breaded and fried	380	5	5	21	190	115
canned with liquid, Snow's, 6½-oz can (drained solids weigh about 2 oz)	90	N.A.	N.A.	<1	N.A.	N.A.
Cod, Atlantic, 3 oz raw	70	<1	<1	<1	N.A.	37
broiled or baked, 3 oz	90	<1	<1	<1	N.A.	47
canned, 3 oz	90	<1	<1	<1	N.A.	47
dried, salted, 3 oz	250	<1	<1	2	18	129
frozen fillets, Mrs. Paul's, 5 oz	110	N.A.	N.A.	2	18	N.A.
Crab, Alaska king, steamed, 3 oz	80	<1	<1	1	10	45
canned blue, 3 oz	80	<1	<1	1	10	76
crab cake, 2 oz	90	<1	1	5	45	90
imitation, from surimi, 3 oz	90	N.A.	N.A.	1	10	17
Crayfish, 3 oz steamed	100	<1	<1	1	10	151
Eel, broiled or baked, 3 oz	200	3	1	13	120	137

*Less than 2% U.S. RDA

Sodium (mg)	Potassium (mg)	Protein (g)	Carbohy-drate (g)	Calcium (% U.S. RDA)	Iron (% U.S. RDA)	Vitamin A (% U.S. RDA)	Vitamin C (% U.S. RDA)
55	260	23	0	*	20	N.A.	N.A.
500	N.A.	17	9	4	20	N.A.	N.A.
90	330	17	0	15	20	N.A.	N.A.
730	110	6	0	4	6	N.A.	N.A.
55	280	15	0	6	6	N.A.	N.A.
105	730	39	0	8	20	*	4
240	300	16	7	4	8	*	*
240	N.A.	4	<1	N.A.	N.A.	N.A.	N.A.
180	N.A.	<1	<1	*	N.A.	N.A.	N.A.
100	570	23	5	8	170	10	N.A.
680	610	27	19	10	170	10	N.A.
1020	120	16	6	4	15	*	*
45	350	15	0	*	2	*	*
65	210	19	0	*	2	*	*
190	450	19	0	*	2	*	*
5970	1240	53	0	15	15	2	6
200	N.A.	22	0	2	2	*	*
910	220	16	0	6	4	*	N.A.
280	320	17	0	8	4	N.A.	N.A.
200	200	12	<1	6	4	N.A.	N.A.
720	75	10	8	*	2	N.A.	N.A.
60	300	20	0	2	20	N.A.	4
55	300	20	0	2	4	60	N.A.

~ FISH & SEAFOOD

	Calories	Saturated fat (g)	Polyunsat-urated fat (g)	Total fat (g)	Calories from fat	Choles-terol (mg)
Flounder fillets, Mrs. Paul's, frozen, 5 oz	110	N.A.	N.A.	2	18	N.A.
Gefilte fish, sweet recipe with broth, 1 piece (1½ oz)	35	<1	<1	<1	N.A.	12
Haddock, 3 oz raw	70	<1	<1	<1	N.A.	49
broiled or baked, 3 oz	100	<1	<1	<1	N.A.	63
frozen, Mrs. Paul's, 5 oz	100	N.A.	N.A.	2	18	N.A.
smoked, 3 oz	100	<1	<1	<1	N.A.	65
Halibut, 3 oz raw	90	<1	<1	2	18	27
broiled or baked, 3 oz	120	<1	<1	3	25	35
Herring, Atlantic, 3 oz raw	130	2	2	8	70	51
broiled or baked, 3 oz	170	2	2	10	90	65
kippered, 1 fillet (1½ oz)	90	1	1	5	45	33
pickled, 1 piece (½ oz)	40	<1	<1	3	25	2
Lobster, 3 oz steamed (½ cup)	80	<1	<1	<1	N.A.	61
Mackerel, 3 oz raw	170	3	4	12	110	60
broiled or baked, 3 oz	220	4	4	15	140	64
canned, drained, ½ cup (3½ oz)	150	2	<1	6	50	75
Monkfish, 3 oz raw	60	N.A.	N.A.	1	10	21
Oysters, raw or steamed, 6 medium (⅓ cup)	60	<1	<1	2	18	46
breaded and fried	170	3	3	11	100	72
canned with liquid, 3 oz	60	<1	<1	2	18	46
Perch, Atlantic, 3 oz raw	80	<1	<1	1	10	36
broiled or baked, 3 oz	100	<1	<1	2	18	46
frozen, Mrs. Paul's, 5 oz	110	N.A.	N.A.	2	18	N.A.
Pike, Northern, 3 oz raw	80	<1	<1	<1	N.A.	33
broiled or baked, 3 oz	100	<1	<1	<1	N.A.	43
Pollock, 3 oz raw	80	<1	<1	<1	N.A.	60
Rainbow trout, 2¼ oz broiled or baked (1 fillet from 1-lb whole fish)	90	<1	1	3	25	45

*Less than 2% U.S. RDA

Sodium (mg)	Potassium (mg)	Protein (g)	Carbohy-drate (g)	Calcium (% U.S. RDA)	Iron (% U.S. RDA)	Vitamin A (% U.S. RDA)	Vitamin C (% U.S. RDA)
210	N.A.	21	5	2	*	*	*
220	40	4	3	*	6	*	*
60	260	16	0	2	6	*	N.A.
75	340	21	0	4	8	*	N.A.
230	N.A.	22	0	*	*	*	*
650	350	21	0	4	8	*	N.A.
45	380	18	0	4	4	2	N.A.
60	490	23	0	6	6	4	N.A.
75	280	15	0	4	6	*	*
100	360	20	0	6	8	*	*
370	180	10	0	4	4	*	*
130	10	2	2	*	*	2	N.A.
320	300	17	1	6	2	*	*
75	270	16	0	*	10	2	*
70	340	20	0	*	8	4	*
360	180	22	0	25	15	8	*
15	N.A.	12	0	*	2	N.A.	N.A.
95	190	6	3	4	35	N.A.	N.A.
370	220	8	10	6	40	*	N.A.
95	200	6	3	4	40	N.A.	N.A.
65	230	16	0	10	6	*	N.A.
80	300	20	0	10	6	*	N.A.
200	N.A.	26	2	2	*	*	*
35	220	16	0	4	4	*	6
40	280	21	0	6	4	*	6
75	300	17	0	6	2	*	N.A.
20	390	16	0	6	10	*	4

~ FISH & SEAFOOD

	Calories	Saturated fat (g)	Polyunsaturated fat (g)	Total fat (g)	Calories from fat	Cholesterol (mg)
Salmon						
pink, 3 oz raw	100	<1	1	3	25	44
canned with bones and liquid, 3 oz (⅓ cup)	120	1	2	5	45	N.A.
red sockeye, 3 oz raw	140	1	2	7	60	53
broiled or baked, 3 oz	180	2	2	9	80	74
canned with bone, drained (3 oz)	130	1	2	6	50	37
Sardines						
canned in oil, drained, 2 sardines (⅘ oz)	50	<1	1	3	25	34
canned in tomato sauce, drained, 1 sardine (1⅓ oz)	70	1	2	5	45	23
Scallops, raw, 6 large or 14 small, 3 oz	80	<1	<1	<1	N.A.	28
breaded and fried, 2 large (1 oz)	70	<1	<1	3	25	19
imitation, from surimi, 3 oz	80	N.A.	N.A.	<1	N.A.	18
Shark, batter fried, 3 oz	190	3	3	12	110	50
Shrimp, 4 large steamed (¾ oz)	20	<1	<1	<1	N.A.	43
breaded and fried, 4 large (1 oz)	70	<1	2	4	35	53
canned, drained, 3 oz (⅔ cup)	100	<1	<1	2	18	147
imitation, from surimi, 3 oz	90	N.A.	N.A.	1	10	31
Smelt, broiled or baked, 3 oz	110	<1	1	3	25	76
Snapper, broiled or baked, 3 oz	110	<1	<1	2	18	40
Sole fillets, Mrs. Paul's, frozen, 5 oz	110	N.A.	N.A.	2	18	N.A.
Squid, 3 oz floured and fried	150	2	2	6	50	221
Surimi (from pollock), 3 oz	80	N.A.	N.A.	<1	N.A.	25
Swordfish, broiled or baked, 3 oz	130	1	1	4	35	43

*Less than 2% U.S. RDA

Sodium (mg)	Potassium (mg)	Protein (g)	Carbohy-drate (g)	Calcium (% U.S. RDA)	Iron (% U.S. RDA)	Vitamin A (% U.S. RDA)	Vitamin C (% U.S. RDA)
55	270	17	0	N.A.	4	2	N.A.
470	280	17	0	20	4	*	*
40	330	18	0	*	2	4	N.A.
55	320	23	0	*	4	4	N.A.
460	320	17	0	20	6	2	*
120	95	6	0	10	4	*	N.A.
160	130	6	0	10	6	2	*
140	270	14	2	2	*	N.A.	N.A.
140	105	6	3	*	2	N.A.	N.A.
680	90	11	9	*	2	N.A.	N.A.
100	130	16	5	4	6	4	N.A.
50	40	5	0	*	4	N.A.	N.A.
105	65	6	3	2	2	N.A.	N.A.
140	180	20	<1	6	15	N.A.	N.A.
600	75	11	8	*	4	N.A.	N.A.
65	320	19	0	6	6	N.A.	N.A.
50	440	22	0	4	*	N.A.	N.A.
170	N.A.	22	0	2	2	*	*
260	240	15	7	4	6	N.A.	6
120	95	13	6	*	*	N.A.	N.A.
100	310	22	0	*	6	2	*

~ FISH & SEAFOOD/ LAMB/ PORK	Calories	Saturated fat (g)	Polyunsat- urated fat (g)	Total fat (g)	Calories from fat	Choles- terol (mg)
Tuna, fresh bluefin, broiled or baked, 3 oz	160	1	2	5	45	42
canned in oil, drained, light, 3 oz	170	1	3	7	60	15
white albacore (unsalted has 45 mg sodium)	160	N.A.	N.A.	7	60	26
canned in water, drained, light, 3 oz	110	<1	<1	<1	N.A.	N.A.
white albacore (unsalted has 45 mg sodium)	120	<1	<1	2	18	35
Leg, roasted, lean and fat, 3 oz	240	9	N.A.	16	140	N.A.
lean only, 3 oz	160	3	N.A.	6	50	N.A.
Loin chop, broiled, lean and fat, 2½ oz	260	12	N.A.	21	190	58
lean only, 1¾ oz	90	2	N.A.	4	35	39
Patty, cooked, 3 oz	230	8	1	16	140	80
Rib chop, broiled, lean and fat, 2⅓ oz	270	13	N.A.	24	220	N.A.
lean only, 1½ oz	90	3	N.A.	5	45	N.A.
Shoulder, roasted, lean and fat, 3 oz	290	13	N.A.	23	210	N.A.
lean only, 3 oz	170	5	N.A.	9	80	N.A.
Bacon						
Canadian, 2 slices cooked (from 2 oz raw)	90	1	<1	4	35	27
cured pork, 3 slices raw (20 per lb)	380	14	5	39	350	46
3 slices cooked	110	3	1	9	80	16
Chitterlings, cooked, 3 oz (from 6½ oz raw)	260	9	6	24	220	122
Ham						
canned chopped, 3 oz	200	5	2	16	140	42
canned whole, roasted, 3 oz	140	2	<1	7	60	34

*Less than 2% U.S. RDA

Sodium (mg)	Potassium (mg)	Protein (g)	Carbohy-drate (g)	Calcium (% U.S. RDA)	Iron (% U.S. RDA)	Vitamin A (% U.S. RDA)	Vitamin C (% U.S. RDA)
45	280	25	0	N.A.	8	45	N.A.
300	180	25	0	*	8	*	N.A.
340	280	23	0	*	4	N.A.	N.A.
300	270	25	0	*	20	N.A.	N.A.
330	240	23	0	N.A.	4	N.A.	N.A.
50	240	22	0	*	10	N.A.	N.A.
60	270	24	0	*	15	N.A.	N.A.
40	180	16	0	*	6	N.A.	N.A.
35	160	14	0	*	6	N.A.	N.A.
55	240	21	0	*	8	*	*
35	150	14	0	*	4	N.A.	N.A.
30	130	12	0	*	6	N.A.	N.A.
45	210	18	0	*	6	N.A.	N.A.
55	260	23	0	*	10	N.A.	N.A.
720	180	11	<1	*	2	*	15
470	95	6	0	*	2	*	2
300	90	6	<1	*	2	*	10
35	5	9	0	2	20	*	*
1160	240	14	<1	*	6	*	2
910	300	18	<1	*	6	*	30

～ PORK/ POULTRY

	Calories	Saturated fat (g)	Polyunsaturated fat (g)	Total fat (g)	Calories from fat	Cholesterol (mg)
cured whole, roasted, lean and fat, 3 oz	210	5	2	14	130	52
lean only, 3 oz	130	2	<1	5	45	47
fresh whole, roasted, lean and fat, 3 oz (⅔ cup)	250	6	2	18	160	79
lean only, 3 oz	190	3	1	9	80	80
Pork fatback, 1 oz	230	9	3	25	230	16
Pork loin						
chop, lean and fat, 3 oz (from 3¾-oz raw)	260	7	2	20	180	74
lean only, 2½ oz	170	3	1	10	90	62
roast, lean and fat, 3 oz	270	8	2	21	190	77
lean only, 3 oz	200	4	1	12	110	77
Pork shoulder roast						
fresh, lean and fat, 3 oz (⅔ cup)	280	8	3	22	200	81
lean only, 3 oz	210	4	2	13	120	82
cured picnic, lean and fat, 3 oz (⅔ cup)	240	7	2	18	160	49
lean only, 3 oz	150	2	<1	6	50	41
Salt pork, cured, 1 oz raw	210	8	3	23	210	25
Spareribs, pork, braised, lean and fat, 3 oz	340	10	3	26	230	103
Bacon, turkey, Louis Rich, 1 slice cooked	35	<1	<1	3	25	9
Chicken, canned chunk style (Swanson), 2½ oz	130	N.A.	N.A.	8	70	N.A.
premium chunk white, 2½ oz	80	N.A.	N.A.	2	18	N.A.
premium white and dark, 2½ oz	100	N.A.	N.A.	4	35	N.A.
Chicken, dark meat						
fried, batter-dipped with skin, 10 oz	830	14	12	52	470	247
without skin, 5 oz (1 cup)	330	4	4	16	140	135

*Less than 2% U.S. RDA

Sodium (mg)	Potassium (mg)	Protein (g)	Carbohy-drate (g)	Calcium (% U.S. RDA)	Iron (% U.S. RDA)	Vitamin A (% U.S. RDA)	Vitamin C (% U.S. RDA)
1010	240	18	0	*	4	*	*
1130	270	21	0	*	6	*	*
50	280	21	0	*	6	*	*
55	320	24	0	*	6	*	*
0	20	<1	0	*	*	*	*
50	260	19	0	*	6	*	*
50	250	19	0	*	6	*	*
55	270	20	0	*	6	*	*
60	310	23	0	*	6	*	*
60	260	19	0	*	8	*	*
65	300	22	0	*	8	*	*
910	220	17	0	*	6	*	*
1050	250	21	0	*	6	*	*
400	20	1	0	*	*	*	*
80	270	25	0	4	10	*	*
210	35	3	<1	*	*	N.A.	N.A.
230	N.A.	14	0	2	6	*	*
250	N.A.	16	1	*	2	*	*
240	N.A.	16	0	*	4	*	*
820	520	61	26	6	25	6	*
135	350	41	4	2	15	2	*

	Calories	Saturated fat (g)	Polyunsaturated fat (g)	Total fat (g)	Calories from fat	Cholesterol (mg)
fried, flour-coated with skin, 6½ oz	520	8	7	31	280	169
roasted with skin, 6 oz	420	7	6	26	230	152
without skin, 5 oz (1 cup)	290	4	3	14	130	130
stewed with skin, 6½ oz	430	8	6	27	240	151
without skin, 5 oz (1 cup)	270	3	3	13	120	123
Chicken, light meat						
fried, batter-dipped with skin, 6½ oz	520	8	7	29	260	157
without skin, 5 oz (1 cup)	270	2	2	8	70	125
fried, flour-coated, with skin, 4½ oz	320	4	4	16	140	113
roasted with skin, 4½ oz	290	4	3	14	130	111
without skin, 5 oz (1 cup)	240	2	1	6	50	118
Duck, domesticated, roasted, 8 oz	450	9	3	25	230	198
Goose, domesticated, roasted, 1⅓ lb	1410	27	9	75	680	569
Turkey						
canned premium chunk, Swanson, 2½ oz, white	90	N.A.	N.A.	2	18	N.A.
white and dark	90	N.A.	N.A.	3	25	N.A.
ground frozen regular, Louis Rich, 15% fat by weight, 1 cooked edible oz (1 lb raw yields 11⅓ oz cooked)	60	1	1	4	35	25
ground fresh lean, Louis Rich, 10% fat by weight, 1 cooked edible oz (1 lb raw yields 12¼ oz cooked)	50	<1	<1	3	25	25
roasted, dark meat, 5 oz (1 cup)	260	3	3	10	90	119
white meat, 5 oz (1 cup)	220	1	1	5	45	97

*Less than 2% U.S. RDA

Sodium (mg)	Potassium (mg)	Protein (g)	Carbohy-drate (g)	Calcium (% U.S. RDA)	Iron (% U.S. RDA)	Vitamin A (% U.S. RDA)	Vitamin C (% U.S. RDA)
160	420	50	8	4	20	4	*
150	370	43	0	2	15	6	*
130	340	38	0	2	15	2	*
130	310	43	0	2	15	6	*
105	250	36	0	2	15	*	*
540	350	44	18	4	15	2	*
115	370	46	<1	2	10	*	*
100	310	40	2	2	10	*	*
100	300	38	0	*	10	2	*
110	350	43	0	2	10	*	*
140	560	52	0	2	40	4	*
450	2290	171	0	8	110	N.A.	*
260	N.A.	16	0	*	2	*	*
280	N.A.	15	1	*	2	*	*
25	80	7	<1	*	4	N.A.	N.A.
30	95	7	<1	*	2	N.A.	N.A.
110	410	40	0	4	20	*	*
90	430	42	0	2	15	*	*

POULTRY/ SAUSAGES & LUNCHEON MEATS	Calories	Saturated fat (g)	Polyunsat-urated fat (g)	Total fat (g)	Calories from fat	Choles-terol (mg)
wing, meat and skin, 6½ oz	430	6	6	23	210	150
Turkey roast, frozen, light and dark, 1 slice (2 oz)	90	N.A.	N.A.	3	25	30
Barbeque loaf, 1 oz	50	<1	<1	3	25	11
Beef loaf, cured, 1 oz	90	3	<1	7	60	18
jellied, 1 oz	30	<1	<1	<1	N.A.	N.A.
Bologna						
beef, 1 slice (1 oz)	90	3	<1	8	70	16
chicken, Weaver, 1 oz	45	N.A.	N.A.	4	35	N.A.
pork, 1 oz	70	2	<1	6	50	17
turkey, Louis Rich, 1 slice (1 oz)	60	2	1	5	45	20
Bratwurst, 1 link cooked (from 3 oz raw)	260	8	2	22	200	51
Braunschweiger (liver sausage), 1 oz	100	3	1	9	80	44
Chicken breast, cold cuts, Weaver, 1 slice hickory smoked, oven roasted	25	N.A.	N.A.	<1	N.A.	N.A.
Chicken roll, light, 2 slices (2 oz)	90	1	<1	4	35	28
Chicken spread						
canned, Underwood, chunky, ½ of 4½-oz can	150	N.A.	N.A.	11	100	35
light, ½ of 4¼-oz can	80	N.A.	N.A.	3	25	N.A.
sandwich salad spread (also turkey salad), 1 tbsp	25	<1	<1	2	18	4
Corned beef spread, Underwood, ½ of 4¼-oz can	120	N.A.	N.A.	10	90	45
Corned beef jellied loaf, 1 oz	45	<1	<1	2	18	13
Dutch loaf, 1 oz	70	2	<1	5	45	13
Frankfurter, 1 frank						
beef, 1½ oz	140	5	<1	13	120	27
beef and pork	140	5	1	13	120	22

*Less than 2% U.S. RDA

324 ~

Sodium (mg)	Potassium (mg)	Protein (g)	Carbohy-drate (g)	Calcium (% U.S. RDA)	Iron (% U.S. RDA)	Vitamin A (% U.S. RDA)	Vitamin C (% U.S. RDA)
115	490	51	0	4	20	*	*
380	170	12	2	*	6	N.A.	N.A.
380	95	5	2	*	2	N.A.	8
380	60	4	<1	*	4	N.A.	6
380	115	5	0	*	6	N.A.	N.A.
280	45	4	<1	*	4	N.A.	10
190	N.A.	2	<1	N.A.	N.A.	N.A.	N.A.
340	80	4	<1	*	*	*	15
240	50	3	<1	2	2	N.A.	N.A.
470	180	12	2	4	8	*	*
320	55	4	<1	*	20	80	4
190	N.A.	4	<1	N.A.	N.A.	N.A.	N.A.
330	130	11	1	2	4	N.A.	N.A.
580	N.A.	10	3	*	4	2	*
300	N.A.	11	2	N.A.	N.A.	N.A.	N.A.
50	25	2	1	*	*	*	*
610	N.A.	6	N.A.	*	8	*	*
270	30	7	0	*	4	N.A.	4
350	105	4	2	2	2	N.A.	8
460	75	5	<1	*	4	N.A.	20
500	75	5	1	*	2	N.A.	20

~ SAUSAGES & LUNCHEON MEATS	Calories	Saturated fat (g)	Polyunsat- urated fat (g)	Total fat (g)	Calories from fat	Choles- terol (mg)
with cheese	140	5	1	12	110	29
chicken	120	3	2	9	80	45
turkey, Louis Rich	100	3	2	8	70	42
Ham and cheese loaf, 1 slice (1 oz)	70	2	<1	6	50	16
Ham, deli, chopped loaf, 1 oz	70	2	<1	5	45	15
deviled spread, Under- wood, ½ of 4¼-oz can	220	N.A.	N.A.	20	180	40
light, ½ of 4¼-oz can	120	N.A.	N.A.	8	70	N.A.
sandwich salad spread, 1 tbsp	30	<1	<1	2	18	6
sliced regular, 11% fat by weight, 1 oz	50	1	<1	3	25	16
sliced extra lean, 5% fat by weight, 1 oz	40	<1	<1	1	10	13
turkey ham, Louis Rich, 1 slice (1 oz)	35	<1	<1	1	10	19
Headcheese, 1 slice (1 oz)	60	1	<1	5	45	23
Honey loaf, 1 oz	40	<1	<1	1	10	10
Kielbasa						
pork, 1 oz	90	3	<1	8	70	20
turkey, Louis Rich, 10% fat by weight, 1 oz	40	<1	<1	2	18	19
Lebanon bologna, 1 oz	60	2	<1	4	35	20
Liverwurst, 1 oz	90	3	<1	8	70	45
Liverwurst spread, Underwood, ½ of 4¼-oz can	180	N.A.	N.A.	15	140	90
Olive loaf, pork, 1 oz	70	2	<1	5	45	11
Pastrami						
beef, 1 oz	100	3	<1	8	70	26
turkey, Louis Rich, 1 slice (1 oz)	30	<1	<1	1	10	18
Pepper loaf, 1 oz	40	<1	<1	2	18	13
Pepperoni, 1 slice (⅕ oz), 1⅜″ diameter, ⅛″ thick	30	<1	<1	2	18	N.A.

*Less than 2% U.S. RDA

Sodium (mg)	Potassium (mg)	Protein (g)	Carbohy-drate (g)	Calcium (% U.S. RDA)	Iron (% U.S. RDA)	Vitamin A (% U.S. RDA)	Vitamin C (% U.S. RDA)
470	90	6	<1	2	4	N.A.	15
620	N.A.	6	3	4	6	N.A.	*
510	85	6	1	6	6	N.A.	N.A.
380	85	5	<1	*	2	N.A.	10
390	90	5	0	*	*	*	10
640	N.A.	9	N.A.	*	6	*	*
250	N.A.	11	2	N.A.	N.A.	N.A.	N.A.
135	20	1	2	*	*	N.A.	*
370	95	5	<1	*	2	*	15
410	100	6	<1	*	*	*	10
300	80	5	<1	*	2	N.A.	N.A.
360	10	5	<1	*	2	*	10
370	95	5	2	*	2	*	10
250	65	4	<1	*	2	*	*
250	55	5	<1	*	2	N.A.	N.A.
380	85	6	<1	*	4	N.A.	10
N.A.	N.A.	4	<1	*	10	N.A.	N.A.
470	N.A.	8	4	*	35	130	*
420	85	3	3	4	*	N.A.	4
350	65	5	<1	*	4	N.A.	*
290	80	5	<1	*	2	N.A.	N.A.
430	110	5	1	*	2	*	10
110	20	1	<1	*	*	N.A.	N.A.

~ SAUSAGES & LUNCHEON MEATS	Calories	Saturated fat (g)	Polyunsaturated fat (g)	Total fat (g)	Calories from fat	Cholesterol (mg)
Pickle and pimento loaf, pork, 1 oz	70	2	<1	6	50	10
Picnic loaf, 1 oz	70	2	<1	5	45	11
Pork luncheon meat, canned, 1 oz	100	3	1	9	80	18
Salami						
beef beerwurst, 1 slice (4" diameter, ⅛" thick)	80	3	<1	7	60	14
hard, pork, 1 slice (⅓ oz)	40	1	<1	3	25	N.A.
pork beerwurst, 1 slice	60	1	<1	4	35	14
smoked beef, 1 oz	70	3	<1	6	50	18
turkey cotto salami, Louis Rich, 1 slice (1 oz)	50	1	1	4	35	22
Sausage						
blood, 1 oz	110	4	1	10	90	34
Italian pork sausage, 1 link cooked, 2⅓ oz (from 3.2 oz raw)	220	6	2	17	150	52
Polish (see Kielbasa, above)						
pork, country-style, 1 link cooked (from 1 oz raw)	50	1	<1	4	35	11
1 patty cooked (from 2 oz raw)	100	3	1	8	70	22
smoked beef, 1 link cooked, 1½ oz	130	5	<1	12	110	29
smoked pork, 1 link cooked, 2⅓ oz (4" long, 1⅛" diameter)	270	8	3	22	200	46
1 little link, ½ oz (2" long, ¾" diameter)	60	2	<1	5	45	11
smoked turkey, Louis Rich, 1 oz	45	<1	<1	2	18	18
summer sausage, 1 oz	100	3	<1	8	70	21
turkey, frozen breakfast sausage (Louis Rich), 1 cooked oz (1 lb yields 13 oz)	60	2	1	4	35	22

*Less than 2% U.S. RDA

Sodium (mg)	Potassium (mg)	Protein (g)	Carbohydrate (g)	Calcium (% U.S. RDA)	Iron (% U.S. RDA)	Vitamin A (% U.S. RDA)	Vitamin C (% U.S. RDA)
390	95	3	2	2	2	N.A.	6
330	75	4	1	*	2	N.A.	8
370	60	4	<1	*	*	*	*
240	40	3	<1	*	2	N.A.	6
230	N.A.	2	<1	*	*	*	*
290	60	3	<1	*	*	*	10
330	65	4	<1	*	4	N.A.	8
270	65	4	<1	*	4	N.A.	N.A.
N.A.	N.A.	4	<1	N.A.	N.A.	N.A.	N.A.
620	200	13	1	*	6	*	2
170	45	3	<1	*	*	*	*
350	95	5	<1	*	2	*	*
490	75	6	1	*	6	N.A.	8
1020	230	15	1	2	6	N.A.	2
240	55	4	<1	*	*	*	*
240	55	5	<1	*	2	N.A.	N.A.
350	75	5	<1	*	4	N.A.	10
210	85	6	<1	*	4	N.A.	N.A.

~ SAUSAGES & LUNCHEON MEATS/ SIMULATEDPRODUCTS	Calories	Saturated fat (g)	Polyunsat- urated fat (g)	Total fat (g)	Calories from fat	Choles- terol (mg)
Vienna sausage, canned, 1 link (7 sausages per can)	50	2	<1	4	35	8
Tuna salad, ½ cup (3½ oz)	190	2	4	10	90	13
Turkey loaf, white meat, 2 slices (1½ oz)	50	<1	<1	<1	N.A.	17
Turkey roll, light, 2 slices (2 oz)	80	1	1	4	35	24
light and dark, 2 oz	80	1	1	4	35	31
Bacon (Worthington Foods), Morningstar Farms break- fast strips, 3 strips	80	1	4	6	50	0
Beef (Worthington Foods), canned savory slices, 2 slices (2 oz)	100	N.A.	N.A.	6	50	0
ground beef (Worthington Foods), granburger soy base, 6 tbsp	110	N.A.	N.A.	1	10	0
Bologna, frozen (Worthington Foods), Bolono, 2 slices (1⅓ oz)	60	0	1	2	18	0
Burger, vegetarian						
canned (Worthington Foods), wheat base, ½ cup	150	1	3	4	35	0
no salt added, ½ cup	160	N.A.	N.A.	6	50	0
frozen (Worthington Foods), soy based, 2¼ oz	180	2	6	12	110	0
mix, grain based (Fantastic Foods), Nature's Burger, 3 oz, original flavor	150	N.A.	N.A.	4	35	N.A.
BBQ flavor, pizza flavor, 3 oz	120	N.A.	N.A.	<1	N.A.	N.A.
mix, tofu burger (Fantastic Foods), 3.4 oz, as prepared with tofu	130	N.A.	N.A.	5	45	N.A.
Chicken						

*Less than 2% U.S. RDA

Sodium (mg)	Potassium (mg)	Protein (g)	Carbohy-drate (g)	Calcium (% U.S. RDA)	Iron (% U.S. RDA)	Vitamin A (% U.S. RDA)	Vitamin C (% U.S. RDA)
150	15	2	<1	*	*	*	*
410	180	16	10	*	8	2	4
610	120	10	0	*	*	*	*
280	140	11	<1	2	4	N.A.	N.A.
330	150	10	1	*	6	N.A.	N.A.
350	20	3	4	*	2	*	*
340	35	8	4	*	2	*	*
700	340	19	7	6	25	*	*
390	60	7	2	2	6	*	*
780	40	19	9	*	10	*	*
500	45	17	9	4	15	*	*
350	50	13	5	4	6	*	*
230	N.A.	7	21	N.A.	N.A.	N.A.	N.A.
420	N.A.	4–5	24	N.A.	N.A.	N.A.	N.A.
310	N.A.	11	14	N.A.	N.A.	N.A.	N.A.

~ SIMULATED PRODUCTS	Calories	Saturated fat (g)	Polyunsaturated fat (g)	Total fat (g)	Calories from fat	Cholesterol (mg)
canned (Worthington Foods), Chik, ½ cup diced or 2 slices (2 oz)	90	N.A.	N.A.	8	70	0
frozen (Worthington Foods), ½ cup diced or 3 slices (3 oz)	190	2	8	13	120	0
Chik Sticks, 1 piece (1⅔ oz)	110	1	4	7	60	0
frozen (Worthington Foods), Morningstar Farms Country Crisps, 3 oz breaded chunks	250	N.A.	N.A.	16	140	0
2½ oz patty	220	2	11	15	140	0
Corned beef (Worthington Foods), frozen, 4 slices (2 oz)	120	1	2	6	50	0
Frankfurter (Worthington Foods), Super Links, 1 link (1⅔ oz)	100	1	5	7	60	0
Veja-links, 2 links (2⅕ oz)	140	N.A.	N.A.	10	90	0
Ham spread (Worthington Foods), Frozen Wham, 3 slices (2⅓ oz)	120	1	5	7	60	0
Salami (Worthington Foods), frozen roll, 2 slices (1½ oz)	90	1	3	5	45	0
Sausage (Worthington Foods), Morningstar Farms breakfast links, 3 links (2⅓ oz)	190	2	8	14	130	0
breakfast patties, 2	190	2	6	12	110	0
canned links (Saucettes), 2 links	140	1	6	9	80	0
Scallops (Worthington Foods), canned vegetable Skallops, ½ cup	90	N.A.	N.A.	2	18	0
no-salt Skallops, ½ cup	80	N.A.	N.A.	1	10	0
Steak (Worthington Foods), canned Prime Stakes, soy based, 1 piece (3¼ oz)	160	N.A.	N.A.	10	90	0

*Less than 2% U.S. RDA

Sodium (mg)	Potassium (mg)	Protein (g)	Carbohy-drate (g)	Calcium (% U.S. RDA)	Iron (% U.S. RDA)	Vitamin A (% U.S. RDA)	Vitamin C (% U.S. RDA)
330	20	4	2	*	4	*	*
680	55	13	5	*	2	*	*
390	85	9	4	2	2	*	*
480	70	8	18	2	4	*	*
620	70	8	13	2	4	*	*
740	75	9	8	*	10	*	*
440	25	7	3	*	4	*	*
330	10	8	4	*	*	*	*
940	115	11	3	*	4	*	*
460	75	8	2	2	6	*	*
500	45	12	3	*	4	*	*
710	20	15	7	2	10	*	2
350	50	10	5	2	10	*	*
430	15	15	4	*	2	*	*
80	5	13	4	*	4	*	*
410	35	10	7	*	6	*	*

~ SIMULATED PRODUCTS/ VARIETY MEATS	Calories	Saturated fat (g)	Polyunsaturated fat (g)	Total fat (g)	Calories from fat	Cholesterol (mg)
Stakelets, frozen soy based, 1 piece (2½ oz)	150	1	4	8	70	0
vegetable steaks, canned wheat base, 2½ pieces (2⅕ oz)	110	N.A.	N.A.	2	18	0
Tuna (Worthington Foods), frozen Tuno, 2 oz	100	1	5	7	60	0
Turkey (Worthington Foods), canned Turkee slices, 2 slices (2¼ oz)	130	N.A.	N.A.	9	80	0
Veal (Worthington Foods), frozen breaded, 2½ oz	230	3	6	14	130	0
Brains, pork, braised, 3 oz	120	2	1	8	70	2169
Feet, pigs', cooked, 2½ oz	140	3	1	9	80	71
cured, pickled, 1 oz	60	2	<1	5	45	26
Heart, pork, braised, 4½ oz	190	2	2	7	60	285
beef, 3 oz	150	1	1	5	45	164
Kidneys						
beef, braised, 3 oz	120	<1	<1	3	25	329
pork, braised, 3 oz	130	1	<1	4	35	408
Liver						
beef, braised, 3 oz	140	2	<1	4	35	331
beef, pan-fried, 3 oz	180	2	2	7	60	410
pork, braised, 3 oz	140	1	<1	4	35	302
Liver pâté, goose, 1 tbsp canned	60	N.A.	N.A.	6	50	20
chicken, 1 tbsp canned	25	N.A.	N.A.	2	18	N.A.
Sweetbreads, pork (pancreas), 3 oz cooked	190	N.A.	N.A.	9	80	268
Tongue						
beef, 3 oz	240	8	<1	18	160	91
pork, 3 oz	230	6	2	16	140	124

*Less than 2% U.S. RDA

Sodium (mg)	Potassium (mg)	Protein (g)	Carbohy-drate (g)	Calcium (% U.S. RDA)	Iron (% U.S. RDA)	Vitamin A (% U.S. RDA)	Vitamin C (% U.S. RDA)
460	105	13	7	4	6	*	*
400	15	17	5	*	15	*	*
310	30	5	3	2	2	*	*
430	25	9	3	*	4	*	*
390	120	14	12	8	15	*	*
75	170	10	0	*	10	*	20
N.A.	N.A.	14	0	4	N.A.	*	*
N.A.	N.A.	4	0	*	N.A.	*	*
45	270	30	<1	*	50	*	4
55	200	25	<1	*	45	N.A.	2
115	150	22	<1	*	40	20	*
70	120	22	0	*	30	4	15
60	200	21	3	*	40	610	30
90	310	23	7	*	35	610	30
40	130	22	3	*	100	310	35
N.A.	N.A.	2	<1	N.A.	N.A.	N.A.	N.A.
N.A.	N.A.	2	<1	*	8	*	2
35	140	24	0	*	15	*	8
50	150	19	<1	*	20	N.A.	*
95	200	21	0	*	30	*	2

~ SOUPS

~ *Listings are divided into Canned Soups (listed by type of soup) and Dry Soups (listed by manufacturer). Values for fiber are available for so few soups that they are not included here. Sugar content is not available.*

~ SOUPS, CANNED

	Calories	Saturated fat (g)	Polyunsaturated fat (g)	Total fat (g)	Calories from fat	Cholesterol (mg)
Bean varieties						
Campbell's (bean with bacon), 1 cup (Special Request contains 540 mg sodium)	120	N.A.	N.A.	4	35	N.A.
Chunky varieties (ham 'n butter bean, old fashioned bean with ham), 1⅓ cups	290	N.A.	N.A.	10	90	N.A.
Progresso (ham and bean), 1¼ cups	180	N.A.	N.A.	2	18	N.A.
Beef varieties						
broth						
Campbell's (bouillon), 1 cup prepared	16	0	0	0	0	N.A.
consommé (with gelatin), 1 cup prepared	25	0	0	0	0	N.A.
Swanson, 1 cup	20	N.A.	N.A.	1	10	N.A.
broth based						
Campbell's (beef, noodle, beefy mushroom, vegetable), 1 cup	70	N.A.	N.A.	3	25	N.A.
Progresso (beef, barley, noodle, vegetable), 1¼ cups	160	N.A.	N.A.	4	35	N.A.
Cheese, Campbell's, cheddar, nacho, 1 cup prepared	120	N.A.	N.A.	8	70	N.A.
Chicken varieties						
broth						
Campbell's, 1 cup	35	N.A.	N.A.	2	18	N.A.
low-sodium, 1⅓ cups	40	N.A.	N.A.	2	18	N.A.
Progresso, 1¼ cups	16	0	0	0	0	10
Swanson, 1 cup	35	N.A.	N.A.	2	18	N.A.
broth based						
Campbell's (alphabet, dumplings,gumbo,noodle, rice, stars), 1 cup prepared (Special Request contains ⅓ less salt)	70	N.A.	N.A.	2	18	N.A.

*Less than 2% U.S. RDA

Sodium (mg)	Potassium (mg)	Protein (g)	Carbohydrate (g)	Calcium (% U.S. RDA)	Iron (% U.S. RDA)	Vitamin A (% U.S. RDA)	Vitamin C (% U.S. RDA)
850	N.A.	6	22	6	10	15	*
1150	N.A.	13	36	8	15	80	10
1130	680	12	30	8	15	100	*
820	N.A.	3	1	*	*	*	*
760	N.A.	4	2	*	2	*	*
830	N.A.	2	0	*	*	*	*
850	N.A.	4	8	*	4	20	2
1250	280	13	16	4	15	35	6
750	N.A.	3	10	6	*	20	4
750	N.A.	1	3	*	*	*	*
70	N.A.	3	2	*	6	*	*
720	210	4	0	*	4	*	*
1000	N.A.	2	2	*	2	*	*
880	N.A.	3	8	*	2	10	*

	Calories	Saturated fat (g)	Polyunsaturated fat (g)	Total fat (g)	Calories from fat	Cholesterol (mg)
low-sodium variety (1⅓ cups, chicken with noodles	160	N.A.	N.A.	5	45	N.A.
chunky varieties (noodle, nuggets, rice, vegetable), 1¼ cups	180	N.A.	N.A.	6	50	N.A.
Clam chowder						
Manhattan style						
Campbell's, 1 cup prepared	70	N.A.	N.A.	2	18	N.A.
Chunky variety, 1⅓ cups	160	N.A.	N.A.	5	45	N.A.
Progresso, 1¼ cups	120	N.A.	N.A.	2	18	N.A.
Snow's, scant cup	70	N.A.	N.A.	2	18	N.A.
New England style						
Campbell's, 1 cup prepared	80	N.A.	N.A.	3	25	N.A.
made with whole milk	150	N.A.	N.A.	7	60	N.A.
Chunky variety, 1⅓ cups	290	N.A.	N.A.	17	150	N.A.
Progresso, 1¼ cups	220	N.A.	N.A.	12	110	N.A.
Snow's, scant cup	140	N.A.	N.A.	6	50	N.A.
Corn chowder						
Progresso, 1¼ cups	200	N.A.	N.A.	10	90	10
Snow's, scant cup	150	N.A.	N.A.	6	50	N.A.
Cream style soups						
Campbell's (asparagus, celery, chicken, mushroom, potato, tomato), 1 cup (tomato provides 40% U.S. RDA for vitamin C) (Special Request contains 530 mg sodium)	100	N.A.	N.A.	5	45	N.A.
Chunky varieties (creamy mushroom, chicken mushroom), 1⅓ cups (chicken mushroom provides 25% U.S. RDA for vitamin A)	290	N.A.	N.A.	23	210	N.A.

*Less than 2% U.S. RDA

Sodium (mg)	Potassium (mg)	Protein (g)	Carbohy- drate (g)	Calcium (% U.S. RDA)	Iron (% U.S. RDA)	Vitamin A (% U.S. RDA)	Vitamin C (% U.S. RDA)
85	N.A.	13	15	2	10	40	4
1050	N.A.	10	19	2	6	85	10
830	N.A.	2	11	2	2	30	8
1230	N.A.	7	24	6	10	120	15
1050	360	8	17	4	10	140	6
630	210	3	9	4	4	40	2
870	N.A.	3	12	2	4	*	2
930	N.A.	7	17	10	4	2	4
1180	N.A.	8	25	6	10	*	10
950	460	8	20	6	6	20	4
670	280	8	13	15	4	2	*
840	400	5	22	*	6	6	10
640	280	5	18	15	2	4	*
820	N.A.	2	11	*	*	6	*
1310	N.A.	8	13	2	10	*	2

~ SOUPS, CANNED	Calories	Saturated fat (g)	Polyunsaturated fat (g)	Total fat (g)	Calories from fat	Cholesterol (mg)
Creamy Natural Gold Label (asparagus, broccoli, cauliflower, potato, spinach), 1 cup prepared	100	N.A.	N.A.	6	50	N.A.
made with whole milk	170	N.A.	N.A.	10	90	N.A.
Progresso (chicken, mushroom), 1¼ cups (chicken variety provides 170% U.S. RDA for vitamin A)	170	N.A.	N.A.	11	100	15
creamy tortellini	240	9	1	16	140	35
Fish chowder						
Campbell's, Chunky, 1⅓ cups	260	N.A.	N.A.	14	130	N.A.
Snow's (fish, seafood), scant cup	130	N.A.	N.A.	6	50	N.A.
French onion, Campbell's, 1 cup prepared	60	N.A.	N.A.	2	18	N.A.
Lentil						
Campbell's Home Cookin', 1¼ cups	150	N.A.	N.A.	1	10	N.A.
Progresso, 1¼ cups	140	N.A.	N.A.	4	35	0
Oyster stew (Campbell's), 1 cup	80	N.A.	N.A.	5	45	N.A.
made with whole milk	150	N.A.	N.A.	9	80	N.A.
Pea and split pea						
Campbell's (green pea with ham & bacon), 1 cup	160	N.A.	N.A.	4	35	N.A.
chunky (split pea with ham), 1⅓ cups	240	N.A.	N.A.	6	50	N.A.
Home Cookin' Ready to Serve, ½ of 19-oz can, split pea with ham	190	N.A.	N.A.	4	35	N.A.
low-sodium, 1⅓ cups, split pea	240	N.A.	N.A.	5	45	N.A.
Progresso (green split pea), 1¼ cups (contains 4.5 grams dietary fiber)	160	N.A.	N.A.	3	25	3

*Less than 2% U.S. RDA

Sodium (mg)	Potassium (mg)	Protein (g)	Carbohy-drate (g)	Calcium (% U.S. RDA)	Iron (% U.S. RDA)	Vitamin A (% U.S. RDA)	Vitamin C (% U.S. RDA)
690	N.A.	1	11	*	2	4	8
740	N.A.	5	16	10	2	6	10
940	230	6	14	2	6	*	*
910	320	5	17	15	8	25	*
1290	N.A.	11	25	6	8	*	4
670	290	9	11	15	2	2	*
900	N.A.	2	9	2	2	*	4
830	N.A.	9	26	4	15	60	6
840	490	10	25	4	25	10	*
830	N.A.	3	5	*	8	*	10
880	N.A.	6	10	10	8	2	10
820	N.A.	8	25	*	10	4	*
1070	N.A.	12	33	2	10	80	10
1090	N.A.	12	26	4	10	40	10
25	N.A.	11	38	4	15	25	8
1050	390	11	27	2	15	2	*

| --- | --- | --- | --- | --- | --- | --- |
split pea with ham, 1¼ cups	170	N.A.	N.A.	4	35	N.A.
Tomato						
Campbell's, 1 cup	90	N.A.	N.A.	2	18	N.A.
made with whole milk, 1 cup	160	N.A.	N.A.	6	50	N.A.
Special Request, 1 cup	90	N.A.	N.A.	2	18	N.A.
low-sodium, 1⅓ cups	180	N.A.	N.A.	5	45	N.A.
Progresso, 1¼ cups	120	N.A.	N.A.	3	25	0
Vegetable						
Campbell's (vegetable, homestyle, minestrone, old fashioned, vegetarian), 1 cup (Special Request vegetable has ⅓ less salt)	70	N.A.	N.A.	2	18	N.A.
chunky varieties (Mediterranean vegetable, minestrone), 1¼ cups	170	N.A.	N.A.	5	45	N.A.
Home Cookin' Ready to Serve (old fashioned vegetable beef, old world minestrone), 1¼ cups	140	N.A.	N.A.	3	25	N.A.
Progresso (minestrone, zesty minestrone, vegetable), 1¼ cups (contains 3.8 grams dietary fiber)	120	N.A.	N.A.	5	45	5
Campbell's						
2 Minute Soup Mix (cup), as prepared, 1 pouch, all varieties	100	N.A.	N.A.	3	25	N.A.
Quality Soup & Recipe Mix, 8 oz (1 cup) prepared						
chicken noodle, chicken rice with white meat, noodle	100	N.A.	N.A.	2	18	N.A.
onion, onion mushroom	50	N.A.	N.A.	1	10	N.A.

*Less than 2% U.S. RDA

Sodium (mg)	Potassium (mg)	Protein (g)	Carbohy-drate (g)	Calcium (% U.S. RDA)	Iron (% U.S. RDA)	Vitamin A (% U.S. RDA)	Vitamin C (% U.S. RDA)
970	400	11	24	4	15	80	4
670	N.A.	1	17	*	2	10	45
730	N.A.	5	22	10	4	10	45
470	N.A.	1	17	*	2	10	40
40	N.A.	3	29	4	6	25	50
1100	400	4	20	2	15	30	*
850	N.A.	3	12	*	4	45	4
960	N.A.	5	25	8	10	100	10
1040	N.A.	8	18	4	8	80	10
1110	330	6	19	4	10	35	4
790	N.A.	4	15	*	2	10	*
790	N.A.	4	17	*	4	*	*
740	N.A.	1	10	*	*	*	*

∼ SOUPS, DRY

	Calories	Saturated fat (g)	Polyunsat- urated fat (g)	Total fat (g)	Calories from fat	Choles- terol (mg)
Fantastic Foods, instant noo- dles and soup (cheddar, curry vegetable, miso, to- mato), 1 pkg	160	N.A.	N.A.	7	60	N.A.
Lipton Cup-a-soup, 1 enve- lope, all varieties	110	N.A.	N.A.	4	35	N.A.
Lite-Line low-sodium bouillon, 1 tsp, beef, chicken	12	N.A.	N.A.	<1	N.A.	N.A.
Ramen soup, 1 cup, all vari- eties	330	N.A.	N.A.	14	130	N.A.
Wyler's instant, 1 tsp or 1 cube, beef, chicken, onion, vegetable (onion contains 670 mg sodium)	8	N.A.	N.A.	<1	N.A.	N.A.

*Less than 2% U.S. RDA

Sodium (mg)	Potassium (mg)	Protein (g)	Carbohy-drate (g)	Calcium (% U.S. RDA)	Iron (% U.S. RDA)	Vitamin A (% U.S. RDA)	Vitamin C (% U.S. RDA)
480	N.A.	6	20	4	6	2	4
740	N.A.	3	15	*	4	8	*
5	580	<1	2	*	*	*	*
1420	N.A.	9	41	4	10	4	25
920	10	<1	1	*	*	*	*

❧VEGETABLES

❧ *Fiber content is listed where available. Values for sugar content are not widely available and so are not included here.*

～ VEGETABLES

	Calories	Saturated fat (g)	Polyunsaturated fat (g)	Total fat (g)	Calories from fat	Cholesterol (mg)
Acorn squash, ½ cup cooked	40	<1	<1	<1	N.A.	0
Alfalfa sprouts, 1 cup	10	<1	<1	<1	N.A.	0
Artichokes, fresh cooked, 1 medium (10½ oz)	50	<1	<1	<1	N.A.	0
frozen hearts, Birds Eye Deluxe, 3 oz	30	0	0	0	0	0
Asparagus, fresh cooked, 4 spears (2 oz)	16	<1	<1	<1	N.A.	0
canned, ½ cup (drained, sodium content is about half)	20	<1	<1	<1	N.A.	0
frozen, ⅓ of 10-oz pkg	25	<1	<1	<1	N.A.	0
Asparagus pilaf (see Entrees & Side Dishes)						
Bamboo shoots, fresh cooked, 1 cup	16	<1	<1	<1	N.A.	0
canned, 1 cup	50	<1	<1	<1	N.A.	0
Beets, fresh cooked, ½ cup	25	<1	<1	<1	N.A.	0
canned, ½ cup (low-sodium pack contains 55 mg sodium)	35	<1	<1	<1	N.A.	0
canned pickled, ½ cup	75	<1	<1	<1	N.A.	0
Beet greens, fresh raw, ½ cup	4	<1	<1	<1	N.A.	0
cooked, ½ cup	20	<1	<1	<1	N.A.	0
Broccoli, fresh raw, ½ cup	12	<1	<1	<1	N.A.	0
cooked, ½ cup	25	<1	<1	<1	N.A.	0
frozen, ⅓ of 10-oz pkg	25	<1	<1	<1	N.A.	0
frozen spears in butter sauce, Birds Eye, 3.3 oz	45	N.A.	N.A.	2	18	5
Brussels sprouts, fresh cooked, ½ cup	30	<1	<1	<1	N.A.	0
frozen, ½ cup	35	<1	<1	<1	N.A.	0
Cabbage, fresh raw, ½ cup shredded, all varieties	8	<1	<1	<1	N.A.	0
cooked, ½ cup	14	<1	<1	<1	N.A.	0

*Less than 2% U.S. RDA

Sodium (mg)	Potassium (mg)	Protein (g)	Carbohy-drate (g)	Dietary Fiber (g)	Calcium (% U.S. RDA)	Iron (% U.S. RDA)	Vitamin A (% U.S. RDA)	Vitamin C (% U.S. RDA)
0	450	<1	9	1.2	*	2	70	15
0	25	1	1	0.7	*	2	*	4
80	320	3	12	N.A.	4	10	4	15
140	210	2	7	3	*	4	2	8
0	190	2	3	1	*	2	10	25
430	190	2	3	2.9	*	4	10	35
0	210	3	5	N.A.	2	4	15	40
5	640	2	2	N.A.	*	2	*	*
20	210	5	8	N.A.	2	6	*	4
40	270	<1	6	2.1	*	4	*	8
320	180	1	8	N.A.	*	6	*	8
300	170	<1	19	N.A.	*	4	*	4
40	100	<1	<1	N.A.	2	4	25	10
170	650	2	4	N.A.	8	10	70	30
10	140	1	2	0.6	2	2	15	70
10	125	2	4	2.3	8	6	20	80
20	150	3	4	2.7	4	4	30	60
320	160	2	5	2	2	2	25	70
15	250	2	7	3.7	2	6	10	80
20	250	3	6	2.5	2	4	10	60
15	85	<1	2	1.2	2	2	10	15
20	200	1	3	2.4	4	4	20	30

～ VEGETABLES

	Calories	Saturated fat (g)	Polyunsaturated fat (g)	Total fat (g)	Calories from fat	Cholesterol (mg)
Carrots, fresh raw, 1 (7½") or ½ cup shredded	30	<1	<1	<1	N.A.	0
canned, ½ cup (drained, sodium content is about half; low-sodium variety contains 50 mg sodium)	30	<1	<1	<1	N.A.	0
fresh cooked, ½ cup	35	<1	<1	<1	N.A.	0
frozen, ⅓ of 10-oz pkg	35	<1	<1	<1	N.A.	0
Carrot juice, Hollywood, canned, 6 oz	80	0	0	0	0	N.A.
Cauliflower, fresh raw, ½ cup	12	<1	<1	<1	N.A.	0
cooked, ½ cup	16	<1	<1	<1	N.A.	0
frozen, ⅓ of 10-oz pkg	25	<1	<1	<1	N.A.	0
frozen with cheese sauce, Birds Eye, 5 oz	130	N.A.	N.A.	7	60	10
Celery, fresh, 1 raw stalk, 7½" or ½ cup diced	8	<1	<1	<1	N.A.	0
cooked, ½ cup	12	<1	<1	<1	N.A.	0
Chard, Swiss, fresh raw, ½ cup	4	<1	<1	<1	N.A.	0
cooked, ½ cup	18	<1	<1	<1	N.A.	0
Chicory greens, raw, ½ cup	20	<1	<1	<1	N.A.	0
Chives, fresh raw, 1 tbsp	2	<1	<1	<1	N.A.	0
freeze-dried, 1 tbsp	2	<1	<1	<1	N.A.	0
Collards, fresh raw, ½ cup	18	<1	<1	<1	N.A.	0
cooked, ½ cup	14	<1	<1	<1	N.A.	0
frozen, ⅓ of 10-oz pkg	30	N.A.	N.A.	<1	N.A.	0
Corn, fresh cooked sweet, 1 ear (6") or ½ cup	90	<1	<1	1	10	0
canned, ½ cup (drained, sodium content is about half; low-sodium variety contains 10 mg sodium)	80	<1	<1	<1	N.A.	0
canned cream style, ½ cup (low-sodium variety contains 10 mg sodium)	90	<1	<1	<1	N.A.	0

*Less than 2% U.S. RDA

Sodium (mg)	Potassium (mg)	Protein (g)	Carbohy-drate (g)	Dietary Fiber (g)	Calcium (% U.S. RDA)	Iron (% U.S. RDA)	Vitamin A (% U.S. RDA)	Vitamin C (% U.S. RDA)
25	210	<1	7	1.6	2	2	360	10
300	210	<1	6	1.4	4	6	320	6
50	180	<1	8	1.5	2	4	380	4
55	170	1	9	1.7	4	4	400	6
170	490	1	17	N.A.	6	8	500	6
5	180	1	3	0.9	*	2	*	60
0	200	1	3	1	*	*	*	60
25	180	2	4	2.4	2	4	*	80
560	240	5	12	2	15	2	40	60
45	140	<1	2	0.5	*	*	*	6
50	270	<1	3	N.A.	2	*	*	6
40	70	<1	<1	N.A.	*	2	10	10
160	480	2	4	N.A.	6	15	60	25
40	380	2	4	N.A.	10	6	70	35
0	10	<1	<1	N.A.	*	*	4	4
N.A.	5	<1	<1	N.A.	*	*	2	2
25	135	2	4	N.A.	10	4	60	35
20	90	1	3	N.A.	8	2	40	15
220	1150	12	29	N.A.	90	35	520	300
15	200	3	21	2.1	*	4	4	8
320	200	3	19	1.7	*	2	4	15
365	170	2	23	N.A.	*	4	2	10

~ VEGETABLES

	Calories	Saturated fat (g)	Polyunsaturated fat (g)	Total fat (g)	Calories from fat	Cholesterol (mg)
frozen, ⅓ of 10-oz pkg	80	<1	<1	<1	N.A.	0
frozen ear, 1 (about 4 oz)	140	<1	<1	1	10	0
frozen baby cobs, Birds Eye Deluxe, 2.6 oz	25	0	0	0	0	0
frozen in butter sauce, Birds Eye, 3.3 oz	90	N.A.	N.A.	2	18	5
Corn fritters, Mrs. Paul's, frozen, 2 fritters	250	N.A.	N.A.	12	110	N.A.
Corn soufflé, Stouffer's, frozen side dish, ⅓ of 12-oz pkg	160	N.A.	N.A.	7	60	N.A.
Cucumber, fresh raw, ½ cup slices	8	<1	<1	<1	N.A.	0
fresh whole, 8¼" long	40	<1	<1	<1	N.A.	0
Custom Cuisine, Birds Eye, frozen, 4.6 oz, all varieties (does not include items added during preparation)	110	N.A.	N.A.	4	35	7
Dandelion greens, fresh raw, ½ cup	14	N.A.	N.A.	<1	N.A.	0
cooked, ½ cup	18	N.A.	N.A.	<1	N.A.	0
Eggplant, cooked, ½ cup cubes	14	<1	<1	<1	N.A.	0
canned (caponata), Progresso, ½ can	70	N.A.	N.A.	4	35	0
frozen Sticks, fried, Mrs. Paul's, 3½ oz	240	N.A.	N.A.	12	110	N.A.
Eggplant parmigiana (see Entrees & Side Dishes)						
Endive, raw, ½ cup	4	<1	<1	<1	N.A.	0
Green beans (green, Italian, yellow), fresh cooked, ½ cup	20	<1	<1	<1	N.A.	0
canned, ½ cup (drained, sodium content is about half; low-sodium variety contains 2 mg sodium)	18	<1	<1	<1	N.A.	0
frozen, ⅓ of 10-oz pkg	30	<1	<1	<1	N.A.	0

*Less than 2% U.S. RDA

Sodium (mg)	Potassium (mg)	Protein (g)	Carbohydrate (g)	Dietary Fiber (g)	Calcium (% U.S. RDA)	Iron (% U.S. RDA)	Vitamin A (% U.S. RDA)	Vitamin C (% U.S. RDA)
0	200	3	20	2.4	*	2	2	10
18	390	4	31	N.A.	*	4	6	15
10	380	2	4	2	*	*	*	6
250	150	2	17	2	*	*	8	6
630	N.A.	4	33	N.A.	2	6	2	2
560	200	5	18	N.A.	6	2	2	4
0	80	<1	2	0.3	*	*	*	4
5	450	2	9	1.5	4	6	2	25
520	240	5	15	1	4	6	80	30
20	110	<1	3	N.A.	6	6	80	15
25	120	1	3	N.A.	8	6	120	15
0	120	<1	3	2	*	*	*	*
260	130	2	4	N.A.	*	6	8	*
610	N.A.	4	29	N.A.	2	8	*	*
5	80	<1	<1	0.5	*	*	10	2
0	190	1	5	1.1	2	6	8	10
440	115	1	4	0.7	2	8	8	8
0	180	2	7	2.7	4	6	10	20

~ VEGETABLES

	Calories	Saturated fat (g)	Polyunsaturated fat (g)	Total fat (g)	Calories from fat	Cholesterol (mg)
Kale, fresh raw, ½ cup	18	<1	<1	<1	N.A.	0
cooked, ½ cup	20	<1	<1	<1	N.A.	0
frozen, ⅓ of 10-oz pkg	25	<1	<1	<1	N.A.	0
Kohlrabi, fresh raw, ½ cup	20	<1	<1	<1	N.A.	0
cooked, ½ cup	25	<1	<1	<1	N.A.	0
Leeks, fresh raw, ¼ cup	16	<1	<1	<1	N.A.	0
cooked, ¼ cup	8	<1	<1	<1	N.A.	0
Lettuce, ½ cup (iceberg, loose-leaf, romaine)	4	<1	<1	<1	N.A.	0
Lima Beans, fresh cooked, 1 cup	210	<1	<1	<1	N.A.	0
canned, ½ cup	90	<1	<1	<1	N.A.	0
frozen baby limas, ⅓ of 10-oz pkg	110	<1	<1	<1	N.A.	0
Mung bean sprouts, fresh, ½ cup	16	<1	<1	<1	N.A.	0
canned, ½ cup	8	<1	<1	<1	N.A.	0
Mushrooms, fresh, ½ cup	10	<1	<1	<1	N.A.	0
cooked, ½ cup	20	<1	<1	<1	N.A.	0
canned, ½ cup	20	<1	<1	<1	N.A.	0
frozen whole, Birds Eye Deluxe, 2.6 oz	20	0	0	0	0	0
frozen breaded, Ore-Ida, 2⅔ oz	140	1	1	8	70	5
shiitake, dried, 4 mushrooms (cooked contain 85 mg potassium)	45	<1	<1	<1	N.A.	0
Mustard greens, fresh, ½ cup	8	<1	<1	<1	N.A.	0
cooked, ½ cup	12	<1	<1	<1	N.A.	0
frozen, ⅓ of 10-oz pkg	20	<1	<1	<1	N.A.	0
Okra, fresh cooked, ½ cup	25	<1	<1	<1	N.A.	0
frozen, ⅓ of 10-oz pkg	30	<1	<1	<1	N.A.	0
frozen breaded, Ore-Ida, 3 oz	170	2	1	10	90	5

*Less than 2% U.S. RDA

Sodium (mg)	Potassium (mg)	Protein (g)	Carbohy-drate (g)	Dietary Fiber (g)	Calcium (% U.S. RDA)	Iron (% U.S. RDA)	Vitamin A (% U.S. RDA)	Vitamin C (% U.S. RDA)
15	150	1	3	N.A.	4	4	60	70
15	150	1	4	N.A.	4	4	100	45
15	320	3	5	3.6	15	6	120	60
15	250	1	4	N.A.	*	2	*	70
15	280	2	6	N.A.	2	2	*	70
5	45	<1	4	0.3	*	4	*	6
0	25	<1	2	N.A.	*	2	*	*
0	65	<1	<1	0.3	*	*	8	6
30	970	12	40	9	6	2	15	30
310	330	6	17	5.2	4	15	4	20
30	430	7	20	3.9	2	10	4	10
0	75	2	3	0.6	*	4	*	10
N.A.	15	<1	1	N.A.	*	*	*	*
0	130	<1	2	0.4	*	2	*	2
0	280	2	4	N.A.	*	10	*	6
N.A.	N.A.	2	4	N.A.	N.A.	4	*	N.A.
0	280	2	4	2	*	6	*	4
520	160	4	14	N.A.	*	8	*	*
0	230	1	11	N.A.	*	2	*	*
5	100	<1	1	N.A.	2	2	30	35
10	140	2	2	N.A.	6	4	40	30
30	160	2	3	N.A.	10	8	100	40
0	260	2	6	N.A.	6	2	10	20
0	200	2	6	4.2	8	4	8	20
670	120	3	17	N.A.	4	4	4	*

	Calories	Saturated fat (g)	Polyunsaturated fat (g)	Total fat (g)	Calories from fat	Cholesterol (mg)
Onions, fresh raw, ½ cup, all varieties	20	<1	<1	<1	N.A.	0
canned, ½ cup	20	<1	<1	<1	N.A.	0
canned French fried, Durkee, ⅙ of 2.8-oz pkg	80	N.A.	N.A.	6	50	N.A.
cooked, ½ cup	30	<1	<1	<1	N.A.	0
dehydrated flakes, ¼ cup	45	<1	<1	<1	N.A.	0
frozen chopped, Ore-Ida, 2 oz	20	<1	<1	<1	N.A.	0
frozen with Cream Sauce, Birds Eye, 5 oz	140	N.A.	N.A.	10	90	0
Onion rings, frozen						
Mrs. Paul's Crispy, 2½ oz	180	N.A.	N.A.	10	90	N.A.
Ore-Ida Onion Ringers, 2 oz	140	1	3	7	60	0
Parsley, fresh, ½ cup	10	<1	<1	<1	N.A.	0
freeze-dried, ¼ cup	4	<1	<1	<1	N.A.	0
Parsnips, ½ cup cooked	60	<1	<1	<1	N.A.	0
Peas, edible pod (see Snow or sugar snap peas, below)						
Peas, green, fresh cooked, ½ cup	70	<1	<1	<1	N.A.	0
canned, ½ cup (drained, sodium content is about half; low-sodium variety contains 2 mg sodium)	60	<1	<1	<1	N.A.	0
frozen, ⅓ of 10-oz pkg	70	<1	<1	<1	N.A.	0
frozen with cream sauce, Birds Eye, 5 oz	180	N.A.	N.A.	11	100	0
Peppers, green, red						
cooked, ½ cup	12	<1	<1	<1	N.A.	0
fresh, sweet raw, ½ cup	12	<1	<1	<1	N.A.	0
frozen, ⅓ of 10-oz pkg	20	<1	<1	<1	N.A.	0
hot chili, fresh, ½ cup	30	<1	<1	<1	N.A.	0
see also Condiments						
Poi, ½ cup	130	<1	<1	<1	N.A.	0

*Less than 2% U.S. RDA

Sodium (mg)	Potassium (mg)	Protein (g)	Carbohy-drate (g)	Dietary Fiber (g)	Calcium (% U.S. RDA)	Iron (% U.S. RDA)	Vitamin A (% U.S. RDA)	Vitamin C (% U.S. RDA)
0	130	<1	5	1.6	4	4	25	25
420	125	1	5	1.2	6	*	N.A.	N.A.
85	50	1	5	N.A.	N.A.	*	*	*
10	160	1	7	1.9	2	*	*	10
0	230	1	12	N.A.	4	*	*	20
10	70	0	4	N.A.	*	*	*	*
400	180	2	12	1	6	2	8	10
270	N.A.	2	20	N.A.	*	4	*	*
180	80	2	18	N.A.	*	2	2	*
10	160	<1	2	4.8	4	15	30	45
5	90	<1	<1	N.A.	*	6	20	4
10	290	1	15	2.1	2	4	*	15
0	220	4	13	3	2	8	10	20
340	110	4	11	2.2	2	10	10	25
105	140	5	13	4.3	2	10	15	30
480	210	5	16	3	6	6	15	10
0	90	<1	3	N.A.	*	4	6	130
0	100	<1	3	0.6	*	4	6	110
5	85	1	4	N.A.	*	4	6	90
5	260	2	7	N.A.	*	6	10	300
15	220	<1	33	N.A.	*	8	*	8

	Calories	Saturated fat (g)	Polyunsaturated fat (g)	Total fat (g)	Calories from fat	Cholesterol (mg)
Potato, baked or microwaved with skin (4½–5″ long, 2½″ diameter)	220	<1	<1	<1	N.A.	0
boiled, ½ cup diced	70	<1	<1	<1	N.A.	0
canned, 1 cup	120	<1	<1	<1	N.A.	0
frozen, small whole, Ore-Ida, 3 oz	70	<1	<1	<1	N.A.	0
Potatoes, cheddared						
Betty Crocker mix, ⅙ pkg, all varieties	140	N.A.	N.A.	5	45	N.A.
Budget Gourmet, frozen side dish, 5½ oz pkg	230	N.A.	N.A.	13	120	35
Budget Gourmet, with broccoli, frozen side dish, 5 oz pkg	130	N.A.	N.A.	4	35	25
Potato chips (see Crackers, Chips & Other Snacks)						
Potato flakes, dehydrated, ½ cup	(360)	<1	<1	<1	N.A.	0
prepared with whole milk and butter, ½ cup	120	4	<1	6	50	15
Potatoes, french fried						
Ore-Ida, frozen, Golden Crinkles and Fries, Homestyle Wedges, 3 oz	120	<1	<1	4	35	0
Crinkle Cuts Lites, 3 oz	90	<1	<1	2	18	0
microwave, 3.5 oz	180	1	1	8	70	0
deep fries, shoestrings, 3 oz	160	1	<1	7	50	0
Tater Tots, 3 oz, regular and flavored	150	1	<1	7	60	0
microwave, 2 oz	120	1	<1	7	60	0
Potatoes au gratin						
Birds Eye for One, frozen, 5.5 oz	240	N.A.	N.A.	13	120	30
Stouffer's frozen side dish, ⅓ of 11½-oz pkg	110	N.A.	N.A.	6	50	N.A.

*Less than 2% U.S. RDA

Sodium (mg)	Potassium (mg)	Protein (g)	Carbohy-drate (g)	Dietary fiber (g)	Calcium (% U.S. RDA)	Iron (% U.S. RDA)	Vitamin A (% U.S. RDA)	Vitamin C (% U.S. RDA)
15	870	5	50	N.A.	2	20	*	50
0	300	2	16	0.9	*	*	*	15
900	730	4	26	N.A.	8	20	*	60
40	360	2	16	N.A.	*	2	*	10
600	290	3	21	N.A.	6	*	4	*
450	N.A.	7	22	N.A.	15	6	*	4
340	N.A.	6	18	N.A.	10	2	4	30
135	660	8	83	N.A.	4	8	*	120
350	250	2	16	N.A.	6	*	4	15
25	350	2	20	N.A.	*	2	*	4
35	290	1	16	N.A.	*	2	*	6
35	310	2	26	N.A.	*	2	*	4
25	280	2	22	N.A.	*	2	*	2
690	200	2	20	N.A.	*	2	*	2
180	120	1	13	N.A.	*	2	*	*
590	400	8	24	1	15	4	6	20
510	260	4	10	N.A.	8	2	*	4

∾ VEGETABLES

	Calories	Saturated fat (g)	Polyunsaturated fat (g)	Total fat (g)	Calories from fat	Cholesterol (mg)
Potatoes, Hash Browns						
Betty Crocker Mix, with onions, ⅙ mix	160	N.A.	N.A.	6	50	N.A.
Ore-Ida, frozen shredded, 3 oz, regular, Southern style	70	<1	<1	<1	N.A.	0
Cheddar Browns, frozen, 3 oz	80	1	<1	2	18	5
microwave, 2 oz	120	1	<1	7	60	0
toaster, 1.75 oz	100	3	<1	6	50	5
Potatoes, scalloped						
Betty Crocker mix, ⅓–⅙ prepared pkg, all varieties	150	N.A.	N.A.	6	50	N.A.
Stouffer's frozen side dish, ⅓ of 11½ oz pkg	90	N.A.	N.A.	4	35	N.A.
Potatoes with sour cream						
Betty Crocker Mix, with chives, ⅙ pkg	140	N.A.	N.A.	5	45	N.A.
Budget Gourmet, new potatoes, frozen side dish, 5 oz pkg	120	N.A.	N.A.	6	50	20
Potatoes, three cheese, Budget Gourmet, frozen side dish, 5¾ oz pkg	230	N.A.	N.A.	11	100	30
Potatoes, twice baked						
Betty Crocker Mix, ⅙ pkg, all varieties	210	N.A.	N.A.	11	100	N.A.
Ore-Ida, frozen, 5 oz, all varieties	220	2	2	10	90	2
Pumpkin, fresh cooked, ½ cup	25	<1	<1	<1	N.A.	0
canned plain, ½ cup	40	<1	<1	<1	N.A.	0
canned pie mix, ½ cup	140	<1	<1	<1	N.A.	0
Radishes, raw, ½ cup slices	10	<1	<1	<1	N.A.	0
Rutabagas, ½ cup cooked	30	<1	<1	<1	N.A.	0
Sauerkraut, canned, ½ cup	20	<1	<1	<1	N.A.	0

*Less than 2% U.S. RDA

Sodium (mg)	Potassium (mg)	Protein (g)	Carbohy-drate (g)	Dietary fiber (g)	Calcium (% U.S. RDA)	Iron (% U.S. RDA)	Vitamin A (% U.S. RDA)	Vitamin C (% U.S. RDA)
460	430	2	24	N.A.	*	2	4	*
35	220	1	16	N.A.	*	*	*	4
420	360	3	14	N.A.	2	2	*	4
180	120	1	13	N.A.	*	2	*	*
285	70	1	12	N.A.	*	2	*	*
550	280	4	21	N.A.	6	2	4	*
420	250	3	11	N.A.	8	2	*	4
520	270	3	21	N.A.	4	2	4	*
300	N.A.	3	15	N.A.	6	4	*	4
410	N.A.	8	25	N.A.	15	2	4	8
590	380	5	20	N.A.	6	4	6	*
470	460	4	27	N.A.	6	6	*	*
0	280	<1	6	0.6	*	4	25	10
5	250	1	10	N.A.	4	10	540	8
280	190	2	36	N.A.	6	10	220	8
15	135	<1	2	0.6	*	*	*	20
15	240	<1	7	N.A.	4	2	*	30
780	200	1	5	N.A.	4	10	*	30

～ VEGETABLES

	Calories	Saturated fat (g)	Polyunsaturated fat (g)	Total fat (g)	Calories from fat	Cholesterol (mg)
Shallots, fresh, 1 tbsp chopped	8	<1	<1	<1	N.A.	0
Snap beans (green, Italian, yellow) (*see* Green beans, above)						
Snow or sugar snap peas, fresh cooked, ½ cup	35	<1	<1	<1	N.A.	0
frozen (Birds Eye Deluxe), 3 oz	35	N.A.	N.A.	0	N.A.	0
Spinach, fresh raw, ½ cup	6	<1	<1	<1	N.A.	0
cooked, ½ cup	20	<1	<1	<1	N.A.	0
canned, ½ cup (drained, sodium content is about half)	20	<1	<1	<1	N.A.	0
frozen, ⅓ of 10-oz pkg	25	<1	<1	<1	N.A.	0
frozen creamed						
Birds Eye Combination, 3 oz	60	N.A.	N.A.	4	35	0
Stouffer's, ½ of 9-oz pkg	170	N.A.	N.A.	14	130	N.A.
Spinach au gratin (Budget Gourmet), frozen side dish, 6-oz pkg	120	N.A.	N.A.	5	45	40
Spinach soufflé (Stouffer's), frozen side dish, ⅓ of 12-oz pkg	140	N.A.	N.A.	9	80	N.A.
Squash, summer (crookneck, scallop, zucchini) (*see* Zucchini, below)						
Squash, winter (acorn, butternut, hubbard, spaghetti) (*see* Acorn squash, above)						
Succotash, canned with creamed corn, ½ cup	100	<1	<1	<1	N.A.	0
canned with whole kernel corn, ½ cup (drained, sodium content is about half)	80	<1	<1	<1	N.A.	0

*Less than 2% U.S. RDA

Sodium (mg)	Potassium (mg)	Protein (g)	Carbohy-drate (g)	Dietary fiber (g)	Calcium (% U.S. RDA)	Iron (% U.S. RDA)	Vitamin A (% U.S. RDA)	Vitamin C (% U.S. RDA)
0	35	<1	2	N.A.	*	*	N.A.	*
0	190	3	6	1.3	4	10	2	60
0	170	2	6	3	4	10	2	30
20	160	<1	1	1.1	2	6	40	15
65	420	3	3	2.4	10	20	150	15
370	270	3	3	1.1	10	15	150	25
70	310	3	4	2	10	15	150	40
310	200	2	5	1	8	6	80	20
380	280	4	7	N.A.	10	6	60	4
410	N.A.	5	14	N.A.	20	6	40	25
500	180	6	8	N.A.	8	6	30	4
330	240	4	23	N.A.	*	4	8	30
280	210	3	18	N.A.	*	4	4	10

～ VEGETABLES

	Calories	Saturated fat (g)	Polyunsat- urated fat (g)	Total fat (g)	Calories from fat	Choles- terol (mg)
frozen, ⅓ of 10-oz pkg	90	<1	<1	<1	N.A.	0
Sugar snap peas (*see* Snow or sugar snap peas, above)						
Sweet potato, fresh cooked, ½ cup	170	<1	<1	<1	N.A.	0
canned vacuum pack, 1 cup	230	<1	<1	<1	N.A.	0
canned syrup pack, 1 cup	210	<1	<1	<1	N.A.	0
frozen, 1 cup	180	<1	<1	<1	N.A.	0
frozen candied (Mrs. Paul's), 4 oz	190	0	0	0	0	N.A.
Tomato, fresh raw, 2½" diameter	25	<1	<1	<1	N.A.	0
cooked, ½ cup	30	<1	<1	<1	N.A.	0
canned, ½ cup (low-sodium pack has 15 mg sodium)	25	<1	<1	<1	N.A.	0
Tomato juice, canned, ½ cup	20	<1	<1	<1	N.A.	0
Tomato paste, 6 oz	140	<1	<1	2	18	0
Tomato puree, canned, 1 cup	100	<1	<1	<1	N.A.	0
Tomato sauce, spaghetti sauce (*see* Condiments)						
Turnips, fresh cooked, ½ cup	14	<1	<1	<1	N.A.	0
frozen, ⅓ of 10-oz pkg	14	<1	<1	<1	N.A.	0
Turnip greens, fresh cooked, ½ cup	16	<1	<1	<1	N.A.	0
canned, ½ cup	18	<1	<1	<1	N.A.	0
frozen, ⅓ of 10-oz pkg	20	<1	<1	<1	N.A.	0
V8 juice (Campbell's), 6 oz, regular, spicy hot	35	0	0	0	0	N.A.
no salt added	40	0	0	0	0	N.A.
Vegetable combinations						
Birds Eye Farm Fresh Mix- tures, 4 oz, all varieties	40	0	0	0	0	0

*Less than 2% U.S. RDA

Sodium (mg)	Potassium (mg)	Protein (g)	Carbohy-drate (g)	Dietary fiber (g)	Calcium (% U.S. RDA)	Iron (% U.S. RDA)	Vitamin A (% U.S. RDA)	Vitamin C (% U.S. RDA)
45	280	4	19	N.A.	*	6	4	15
20	300	3	40	4	4	6	560	45
135	800	4	54	N.A.	6	15	410	110
90	400	3	49	2.4	4	15	270	40
15	660	3	41	4	6	6	580	25
60	N.A.	1	47	N.A.	2	4	100	25
10	250	1	5	1	*	4	30	35
15	310	1	7	N.A.	*	4	30	40
200	270	1	5	0.8	4	4	15	30
440	270	<1	5	N.A.	*	4	15	35
110	1590	6	32	N.A.	6	35	80	120
50	1050	4	25	N.A.	4	15	70	150
40	105	<1	4	4.4	*	*	*	15
25	130	3	8	N.A.	6	15	*	20
20	150	<1	3	N.A.	10	4	80	35
330	170	2	3	N.A.	15	10	80	30
10	170	2	3	N.A.	10	10	120	40
600	N.A.	1	8	N.A.	2	4	45	50
45	N.A.	1	9	N.A.	2	4	45	50
25	230	2	8	2.9	4	4	100	60

	Calories	Saturated fat (g)	Polyunsaturated fat (g)	Total fat (g)	Calories from fat	Cholesterol (mg)
Birds Eye International, 3.3 oz (Italian, Japanese, New England, Oriental, pasta primavera, San Francisco)	100	N.A.	N.A.	5	45	0
Vegetable medley, breaded (Ore-Ida), frozen, 3 oz	160	2	1	9	80	5
Vegetables, mixed, canned, ½ cup (drained, sodium content is about half)	45	<1	<1	<1	N.A.	0
frozen, ⅓ of 10-oz pkg	70	<1	<1	<1	N.A.	0
Vegetables in pastry (Pepperidge Farm), frozen, 1 pastry, all varieties	240	N.A.	N.A.	16	140	N.A.
Vegetables, stew (Ore-Ida), frozen, 3 oz	60	<1	<1	<1	N.A.	0
Vegetables, stir fry (Birds Eye), 3.3 oz Chinese style, Japanese style	35	0	0	0	0	0
Water chestnuts, ½ cup canned	35	N.A.	N.A.	<1	N.A.	0
Watercress, ½ cup raw	2	<1	<1	<1	N.A.	0
Yams, ½ cup cooked	80	<1	<1	<1	N.A.	0
Yellow wax beans (see Green beans, above)						
Zucchini, cooked, ½ cup	18	<1	<1	<1	N.A.	0
canned Italian style (Progresso), ½ cup	50	<1	<1	2	18	<1
frozen breaded (Ore-Ida), 3 oz	150	2	1	9	80	5
frozen sticks, light batter (Mrs. Paul's), 3 oz	200	N.A.	N.A.	12	110	N.A.

*Less than 2% U.S. RDA

Sodium (mg)	Potassium (mg)	Protein (g)	Carbohy- drate (g)	Dietary fiber (g)	Calcium (% U.S. RDA)	Iron (% U.S. RDA)	Vitamin A (% U.S. RDA)	Vitamin C (% U.S. RDA)
400	140	3	11	1.7	4	4	25	25
500	180	3	17	N.A.	*	2	20	4
270	170	2	9	2	2	6	120	8
45	200	3	13	2.2	2	6	100	15
340	N.A.	5	19	N.A.	6	8	6	15
50	200	1	11	N.A.	*	2	45	8
530	200	2	8	2	4	6	35	35
5	80	<1	9	N.A.	*	4	*	*
5	55	<1	<1	0.3	2	*	15	10
5	460	1	19	0.7	*	2	*	15
0	170	<1	4	1.4	2	2	6	8
540	330	1	8	2	2	4	6	20
445	150	3	15	N.A.	*	6	2	*
440	N.A.	2	21	N.A.	2	6	*	*

∾ BIBLIOGRAPHY

MAJOR SOURCES OF DATA

Agriculture Handbook No. 8, Revised, Composition of Foods, Raw, Processed, Prepared, U.S. Department of Agriculture, Washington, D.C.

8-1	*Dairy and Egg Products,* 1976
8-4	*Fats and Oils,* 1979
8-5	*Poultry Products,* 1979
8-6	*Soups, Sauces and Gravies,* 1980
8-7	*Sausages and Luncheon Meats,* 1980
8-9	*Fruits and Fruit Juices,* 1982
8-10	*Pork Products,* 1983
8-11	*Vegetables,* 1984
8-12	*Nuts and Seed Products,* 1984
8-13	*Beef Products,* 1986
8-14	*Beverages,* 1986
8-15	*Finfish and Shellfish,* 1987
8-16	*Legumes,* 1986
8-20	*Cereal Grains and Pasta,* 1989

ADDITIONAL REFERENCES

Anderson, James W., M.D. *Plant Fiber in Foods.* HCF Nutrition Research Foundation, Inc., P.O. Box 22124, Lexington, KY 40522, 1990.

Anderson, J.W., and Bridges, S.R. "Dietary Fiber Content of Selected Foods." *American Journal of Clinical Nutrition* 47 (1988): 440–47.

Bowes & Church's Food Values of Portions Commonly Used, 15th ed., revised by Jean A. T. Pennington, Ph.D., R.D. New York: Harper & Row, 1989.

Englyst, H.N.; Bingham, S.A.; Runswick, S.A.; Collinson, E.; and Cummings, J.H. "Dietary Fibre (Non-starch Polysaccharides) in Fruit, Vegetables, and Nuts." *Journal of Human Nutrition and Dietetics* 1 (1988): 247–86.

Leveille, Zabik and Morgan. *Nutrients in Foods.* Cambridge, Mass.: The Nutrition Guild, 1983.

U.S. Food and Drug Administration. "Nutritional Labeling of Food." *Code of Federal Regulations,* Title 21, Parts 100–169, April 1990.

Information was also provided by individual manufacturers and food labels.